HAW

ILLUSTRATED ELEMENTS

HERBALISM

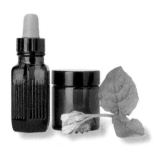

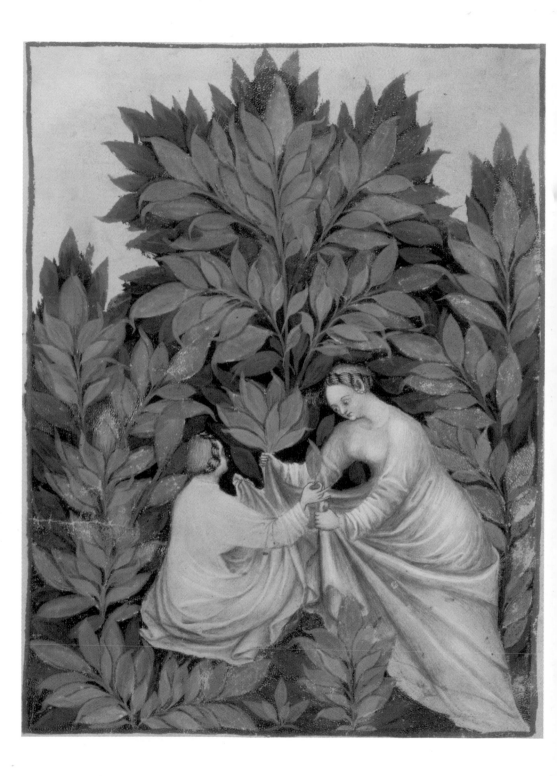

ILLUSTRATED ELEMENTS OF
HERBALISM

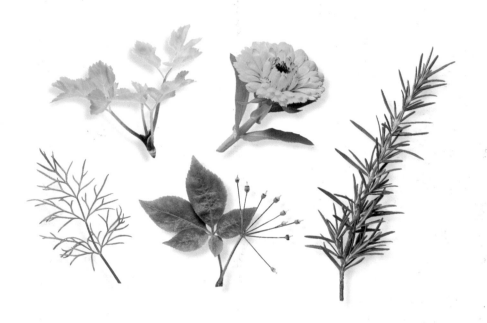

NON SHAW

ELEMENT

First published in Great Britain in 1998 by
ELEMENT BOOKS LIMITED

This edition published 2002 by Element
An Imprint of HarperCollins*Publishers*
77–85 Fulham Palace Road, Hammersmith, London W6 8JB

Element™ is a trademark of HarperCollins*Publishers*

2 4 6 8 10 9 7 5 3 1

NOTE FROM THE PUBLISHER
*Any information given in this book is not intended to be taken
as a replacement for medical advice. Any person with a condition
requiring medical attention should consult a qualified
practitioner or therapist.*

Designed and created with
THE BRIDGEWATER BOOK COMPANY LIMITED

Printed and bound in Hong Kong by Printing Express

British Library Cataloguing in Publication
data available

Library of Congress Cataloging-in-Publication
data available

ISBN 0-00-713602-1

Acknowledgements
Phillip Auchinvole, Clare Bayes, Roger Cooper, Kate Davis, Geoffrey
Gardener, Annette Gerlin, Sam Hollingdale, Barbara Price,
Anna Spyropolous, Julie Spyropolous, Helen Tookey, Charlotte Walsh,
Amelia Whitelaw, Gabriel Whitelaw, Robert Whitelaw

Dedicated to my parents, Joy and Peter Shaw

Picture credits

AKG, London: 14t.
A-Z Botanical Collection: 80c, 82c.
Bridgeman Art Library: 6r (Royal Albert
Memorial Museum, Exeter);
34b (Stapleton Collection);
39b (Archaeological Museum, Heraklion);
67b (Museum Fine Arts, Budapest);
79T (Kunsthistorisches Museum, Vienna);
83t (Russel Cotes Art Gallery & Museum,
Bournemouth); 99b (Musée Crozatier, Le
Puy en Velay). *Corbis-Bettmann*: 37t.
e. t. archive: 2, 8r, 11t, 14b, 15t, 36b, 42tl,
66cr, 73t, 75t, 85b, 101b, 105t, 105b.
Garden Picture Library: 16r (Christopher
Gallagher); 23t (John Glover);
58t (Brigitte Thomas). *Harry Smith
Collection*: 48r, 50b, 76b, 88cr, 104cr.
Image Bank: 22l, 46b, 49b, 102cr, 113r,
129r, 133t. *NHPA*: 64br. *Robert Harding
Library*: 92cr. *Science Photo Library*: 63 .
Stock Market: 60b, 70b, 132l. *Zefa*: 41b.

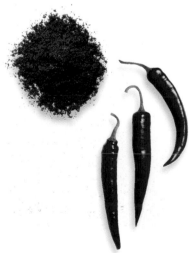

Contents

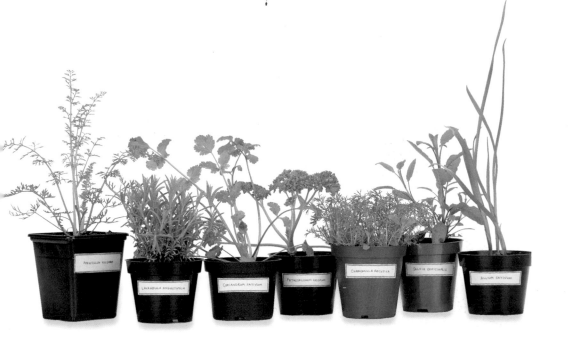

Preface

Herbalism or herbal medicine – the use of plants for healing – is one of the oldest and most widespread of medical therapies, extending back to the earliest times. Every culture has evolved its own traditions of folk medicine, with remedies and rituals using locally available plants. This knowledge was passed orally from parent to child, each generation building on the knowledge of the previous one, until finally this lore was transcribed into manuscripts and printed texts. In this book I hope to continue the tradition by sharing what I have learned in my studies and practice.

ABOVE *Herbs, such as marigold, can be used to make a wide variety of healing remedies.*

Herbalism holds a great attraction for those seeking a more natural, holistic approach to their well-being. Herbalism is a science and an art, combining the objectivity of science with the subjectivity of human experience. It has an holistic view of the world and the body, and is based on an understanding of the interdependence of all things.

This book is a guide to the theory and ideas of professional herbalism, and to its safe home practice. It tells you how herbalism works, and how to grow, make, and use plant remedies at home. While herbs form the basis of much modern pharmacology, the active ingredient is separated from the plant to make the drug. Herbalism, on the other hand, uses the whole plant; its smell, taste, and the way it is used – as a tea, a compress, or tincture, for example – are all important aspects of herbalism. To pick a plant, run your fingers through it, and assault your senses with the aromas released from its leaves, is in itself a therapeutic experience. To be able to make remedies from those plants that will increase and enhance the health and well-being of friends and family is extremely satisfying indeed.

ABOVE *Each ancient culture devised a complete system of herbal medicine.*

BELOW *This book tells you how to use plant remedies at home.*

How to Use This Book

This is a practical book for the general reader who wishes to understand and practice herbalism. It explores the history of herbalism, tells you how herbs work, advises on the best places to find herbs, and how best to prepare them for use. The extensive Materia Medica, is a comprehensive guide to many of the major plants used in herbal medicines. The final sections of the book give wide-ranging information on treating common ailments at home. However, this book is not intended as a lay version of professional medical herbalism and as a general rule does not encourage diagnosis.

BELOW **The Materia Medica section, which gives details of 36 herbs, forms the main part of this beautifully illustrated book.**

A home use box gives suggestions on how best to use the particular herb illustrated.

BELOW **As well as discussing the origins and history of herbalism, the first part of the book shows you how to make herbal preparations.**

Learn how to make tinctures, herbal wines, or fruit vinegars for daily home use.

Clear and concise information on the chemical constituents of herbs.

Anatomical drawings illustrate the particular body system under discussion.

RIGHT **The last part of the book lists common ailments and gives suggestions on which herb to use in their treatment.**

This section details a variety of common ailments and lists herbal preparations that may help to relieve the symptoms.

As well as herbal remedies, other measures, such as diet and exercise, are suggested.

What is Herbalism?

HERBALISM IS *the use of plants to create medicines and remedies for health problems and to enhance well-being. Its main purpose is to stimulate the body's own natural powers of healing by rebalancing and cleansing. Many herbs share the properties of the synthetic drugs of orthodox medicine, but unlike synthetic drugs they are able to restore health without unwanted side effects and without damaging the natural equilibrium of the body. As well as being effective, they are also inexpensive and easy to use.*

ABOVE *Herbs have many of the properties of orthodox drugs but without the side effects.*

Plants have always been used for medical purposes, as well as for food, drink, warmth, shade and shelter, clothing, tools, and dyes. The need for, and exploitation of, plant products have driven and shaped cultures and societies. For example, spice was the enticement that led to the discovery of the New World, and every ship set sail with a botanist to take cuttings and bring them back across the oceans to Europe. The knowledge and control of plants equated with power and riches. New plants generated great wealth for some people and the history of medicinal plants and drugs reflects the same human mixture of altruism and greed.

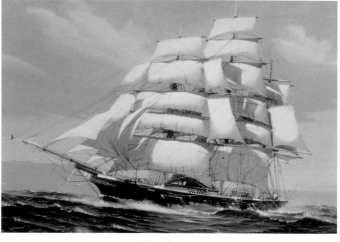

ABOVE *The 16th-century explorers of the New World brought back many new medicinal plants to Europe.*

RIGHT *Throughout the centuries, plants have been exploited for a multitude of purposes, including medicinal and domestic uses.*

Herbalism is the oldest form of medicine and has been in continual use by humankind since prehistoric times. It incorporates a vast amount of learning and experience that overlaps several scientific disciplines. The practice of herbal medicine involves an extensive knowledge of plants, of people and their ailments, together with a special understanding and awareness of what occurs when people and certain plants interact, both generally and chemically.

Herbal medicine incorporates all the hard and soft sciences in its usage – for example, anatomy, chemistry, biology, physiology, pharmacology, pharmacognosy, pathology, and psychology.

You may not realize it, but you are practicing the skills of a herbalist every day. For example, when you are asked "coffee or tea?", you are choosing between two herbal preparations: a filtrate of roasted fruit or an infusion of fermented leaves. Your reply will depend on several factors, including the constitutional state of your body at the time (you may be dehydrated or tired), what it has just done, and what it is about to do (go for a run or go to sleep). The physiological effects of the drink are juggled with internal, external, and personal factors. As you gather this information, you are prioritizing, analyzing, and processing your needs. In a fraction of a second, you have the answer: "I think I would like tea, please!" This is complex reasoning, practiced so often as to appear almost intuitive. These are the skills of the herbalist and the skills encouraged in this book.

A herbalist takes these skills and builds on them over many years, honing them into a seamless system of medicine, based on a knowledge not only of a particular plant but also its effect on a particular individual. In this book it is not necessary to learn all the sciences, but to appreciate them and to be aware of the difference between home and professional practice.

HERBAL MEDICINE TODAY

By the 20th century, chemically manufactured drugs had become dominant throughout the European and the US medical systems, and the use of traditional herbal remedies had declined.

It is only relatively recently that there has been a widespread revival of interest in herbal medicine, and nowadays the World Health Organization (W.H.O.) encourages all countries to protect and cherish their own traditions. Some countries are trying to formalize the learning of, and register the practice of, their herbal knowledge, although it is not easy. Social, political and financial considerations greatly influence all healthcare decisions.

Medical herbalists and native healers in almost every country of the world are striving to retain the integrity and independence of their profession, and the independence and rights of their patients. All professional herbalists, irrespective of country and tradition, undergo a prolonged training, apprenticeship, or initiation. Consultations will be different, but whatever the differences, all herbalists try to practice with the best interests of their patients at heart.

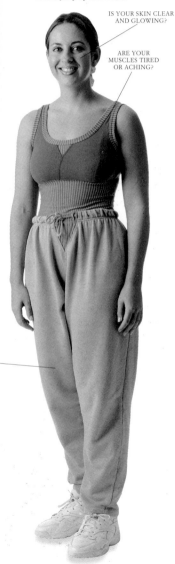

BELOW *Listen to your body, and you will begin to pick up the intuitive skills used so successfully by herbalists.*

IS YOUR SKIN CLEAR AND GLOWING?

ARE YOUR MUSCLES TIRED OR ACHING?

DO YOU FEEL HEALTHY AND ACTIVE?

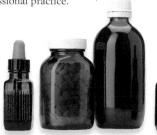

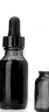

BELOW *Professional herbalists must undergo stringent training before they can prescribe remedies.*

The Origins of Herbal Medicine

FOR MOST OF THEIR EXISTENCE, *human beings have had various but limited resources for treating injuries and diseases. For thousands of years, sickness was blamed on supernatural forces, and treatments included the use of magic, music, prayer, and incantations, as well as crude operations, physical therapy such as diet, fresh air, and exercise, and internal and external remedies based on plants.*

ABOVE *Exercise, particularly meditative forms such as yoga, play a vital role in medical systems around the world.*

In about 500 B.C.E. this supernatural view of disease was displaced by a belief in health as a balance of forces within the body, and disease as a disturbance of that balance. This view did not change the role of herbs in medicine, and plant remedies continued to be used therapeutically. They became an important means of treating illness, as they were seen as a way of restoring balance and harmony to the body.

Throughout the world there developed many different healing systems based on this idea of balancing natural forces, and relying on the medicinal use of plants. These include the Indian system of Ayurveda, the ancient Chinese and the Native American systems, as well as the system of folk medicine which developed in Europe. Each country or culture developed its own tradition and pharmacy from locally growing plants. China and India have the oldest written traditions, dating from about 1000 B.C.E.

Whereas the Indian and Chinese systems still survive today, in Europe the idea of balanced forces within the body gradually disappeared. From the 16th century onward, European cultures expanded into the New World, and medical imperialism made Western medicine the dominant ideal throughout the world, although not necessarily the dominant practice. Many indigenous systems have been deeply affected by this. Although in some countries, such as China, tradition has always been honored and traditional herbal and modern Western medicine are practiced side by side, in other countries "bush" or folk medicine was despised, ignored, or even outlawed as politically dangerous. Local healers and wise women, many of whom held valuable information and skills, were vilified and persecuted.

1600 B.C.E	1000 B.C.E.	800 B.C.E	460–377 B.C.E.	C.E. 100
The Egyptians record the use of herbal medicine on papyri. Herbs mentioned include cilantro, juniper, fennel, thyme, and juniper.	*The Yellow Emperor's Book of Internal Medicine*, the classic work on Chinese traditional medicine. Its central tenet is the idea of the five elements in nature: wood, fire, earth, metal, and water.	The *Atharva Veda* is written. This work details the Indian Ayurvedic tradition of healing using herbs and diet to restore equilibrium in the body.	Hippocrates, the father of medicine, recommends many herbal remedies for his patients including camomile, garlic, cinnamon, and rosemary.	Pedanius Dioscorides writes his *De Materia Medica*, this work describes some of the herbal actions that are known to us today.

CHINA

The oldest medical text in China is *The Yellow Emperor's Book of Internal Medicine*, which is about 3,000 years old and still consulted today. Traditional Chinese medicine is based on the five elements of wood, water, fire, earth, and metal. These elements differ from the European medieval model in that they are not discrete like the four humors (*see p.12*) but linked energetically, constantly interacting and feeding, hindering, or flowing through one another.

Each element is linked to one or more organs, an emotion, a taste, and a season. Specific herbs of the right taste will strengthen the element. For example, the element of earth is related to the stomach and spleen, the emotion is worry, the season is summer, and the taste sweet. A tonic for this element would be the sweet root of licorice, warming and nourishing.

INDIA

India's Ayurvedic medical system, dating back thousands of years, is a plant-based and holistic form of healing. The Sanskrit word Ayurveda

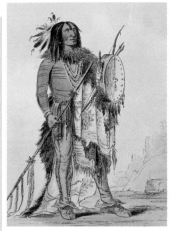

ABOVE *In the North American tradition, the shaman was also the philosopher, wise person, counselor, judge, and storyteller.*

derives from two words meaning "life" and "knowledge." It is not medicine in the Western sense but a way of life, a way to live in harmony with the balance of one's elements and the *prana* or breath of life.

Everyone is made up of the three humors, air (*vata*), fire (*pitta*), and water (*kapha*), the dominant one dictating a person's constitution. Before making a diagnosis the practitioner will assess your humor. Treatment includes the prescription of herbs as well as food, fasting,

spiritual practices, and breathing. Exercises such as yoga, may be recommended and sexual activity or abstinence advised to rebalance excesses or deficiencies.

NORTH AMERICA

In many North American tribes the priest or shaman was also the "medicine man." The world was thought to be pervaded by good and evil spirits that only the shaman could influence, and this meant that he alone could cure disease, perhaps by journeying far in dreams or trances. Drums, rattles, dances, herbs, and sacred plants were also used. Sometimes a trance-inducing sweat lodge was also part of the ritual. This was like a sauna; a special tent was made incredibly hot and used for ceremonial cleansing, both emotional and physical. Fumigation by burning herbs was also practiced. The person would either pass through the fumes or have the smoke blown around the naked body. Medicine animals protected the eight directions of American Indian belief, to give guidance. For example, the eagle came from the east, sharp-eyed and wise.

C.E. 137–199	C.E. 980–1037	C.E. 1493–1541	C.E. 1616–54	C.E. 1769–1843
Claudius Galenus, court physician to Emperor Marcus Aurelius, formalizes the theories of the humors. His books become standardized medical texts.	The great Arab physician Avicenna keeps alive the galenical principles of medicine with his classic work, the *Qanun*. His work influences medical treatment throughout the world.	Paracelsus bases his theories on the Doctrine of Signatures. He predicts the discovery of active ingredients in plants.	Nicholas Culpeper translates the *Pharmacopoeia* into English so that the common people can discover herbal remedies for themselves.	Samuel Thompson learns Native American herbal lore. His books become extremely popular in the U.S.

The Theories of Early Medicine

*Since ancient times, humankind has sought to understand the workings
of the body, the causes of illnesses, and their remedies. Through the ages,
medical practitioners have devised various theories of the human body and
how it works, relating physical and emotional conditions to such things
as the elements and the influence of the planets, and explaining the curative
properties of plants in terms of their appearance or the effects that they produce.*

THE FOUR HUMORS

The system of humors was used to explain the body from ancient Greek times until the study of the anatomy of the body began in the 16th century. According to this system, the human body was made up of four humors or bodily fluids, each one of which was associated with one of the four elements, and responsible for the emotional and physical balance of the individual. Imbalance of the humors brought disease. Balance could be corrected by diet, change of climate, activity, sex, and herbal remedies.

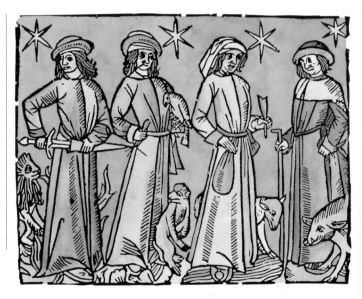

RIGHT *A 16-century depiction of the four humors – it was believed that good health depended on balance of the humors.*

CHARACTERISTICS OF THE FOUR HUMORS

This system made intuitive sense to people; organs could be hot or cold, empty or full, and the diagnosis was literal and descriptive. Patients still use language from the system of humors to describe temperaments, subjective feelings, and symptoms.

Phlegm – found in the lungs and brain. A phlegmatic person is watery. Phlegm is dominant in winter.
Blood – found in the heart and arteries. A sanguine person is airy. Blood is bountiful in the spring.

Black bile or melancholy – found in the spleen. A melancholic person is dry and down to earth. The fall is the most melancholic season.
Choler or yellow bile – found in the gall bladder. A choleric person is fiery and is at their best during the summer.

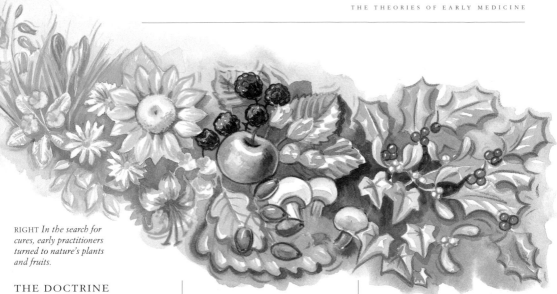

RIGHT *In the search for cures, early practitioners turned to nature's plants and fruits.*

THE DOCTRINE OF SIGNATURES

Based on observation, the Doctrine of Signatures was acknowledged from earliest times and used in herbal medicine throughout the Middle Ages. The doctrine holds that natural remedies have visual clues for their use – that is to say the use of a plant is obvious from its appearance and structure. For example, yellow herbs are good for the yellow bile of the liver; wound-healing plants such as comfrey and plantain have shield-like leaves.The wrinkled fruit of the walnut was eaten to strengthen the brain.

According to this system one plant could have several uses. The dandelion, for example, has yellow flowers that bring sunshine to the liver; its tubular flower stems, like pipes, stimulate water; the rippling wave-like leaves direct excess water away from the body; and the solid, earthy taproot builds up and nourishes the liver.

The 16th-century physician Paracelsus based his theories (*see p.15*) around the doctrine.

ASTROLOGY

Nicholas Culpeper (1616–54) was an astrologer-physician: he believed it impossible to attempt to heal a patient without taking note of planetary influences. As each part of the body was ruled by a different planet – e.g., the heart by the Sun,

HERBS AND THEIR PLANETS

Herbs were assigned to planets according to their active properties:
Sun: angelica, marigold. Hot, generous, radiating plants
Moon: cucumber, cabbages, chickweed. Cooling plants
Mars: tobacco, garlic. Hot and biting plants
Venus: thyme, elderflower. Warm and nourishing plants
Mercury: parsley, elecampane. Mercurial, messenger-carrying herbs and alteratives
Jupiter: dandelion, dock. Jovial, strengthening, liver-balancing herbs
Saturn: comfrey and horsetail. Holding and strengthening plants

the genitals by Venus, and the bones by Saturn – it was necessary for a doctor to study astrology.

A chart was drawn up by the physician at the onset of a person's illness, to determine the planetary positions and from these the best type of treatment.

SYMPATHY AND ANTIPATHY

This theory has many practical applications that are still in use today. Remedies were applied according to very simple rules. Treatment by sympathy, or like-to-like, meant that a patient with a slight fever would be kept warm and given warm, stimulant herbs such as hot ginger and sage tea. These would encourage the circulation and induce sweating. Alternatively, the patient could be given treatment by antipathy, or like-to-unlike. In this case, the patient would be given cooling washes to help reduce his temperature, as well as cool, eliminating herbs such as chickweed or cleavers.

History of Western Herbalism

Western herbalism has a long and noble, though often troubled, history. On one hand it can be seen as a steadily developing science, with each age building upon the wisdom of earlier physicians. On the other, as a homely craft with its roots in traditional wisdom, it has at times appeared to threaten the power of established medicine.

THE ANCIENT WORLD

The Greek physician Hippocrates (460–377 B.C.E.) is honored as the father of modern medicine. He considered all the factors that promoted health, even altitude and weather, and recommended diet, hygiene, and herbs. The first European treatise on the properties and uses of medicinal plants, *De Materia Medica*, was compiled by Pedanius Dioscorides in C.E. 100.

Galen (C.E. 131–199) was a Greek military physician who learned much while accompanying soldiers on campaigns. He formalized the theory of humors (*see p. 12*). His ideas and practical treatment, known as Galenic medicine, became a standard text and practice for hundreds of years, throughout the Middle Ages.

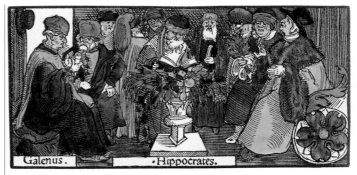

ABOVE *The works of Hippocrates and Galen dominated Western medical practice for centuries.*

THE MIDDLE AGES

During the Crusades of the 11th to the 13th centuries, Europeans came into contact with the writings of the Arab practitioner Avicenna (C.E. 980–1037). His medical work *Qanun* stimulated new ideas that spread to the first medical school of medieval Europe in Salerno, Italy, and from there throughout the rest of Europe.

One of the most famous herbalists of this period was Hildegard of Bingen. Born in 1098, Hildegard was the Abbess of Bingen in Germany, where she used music, art, contemplation, diet, herbs, and prayer to calm and heal. She wrote two herbals and like herbalists today, Hildegard did not separate mind and body but applied her herbal remedies compassionately, to the whole person.

In the Middle Ages herbalism was a dangerous profession for women, regardless of whether their patients died or survived. Their efforts were considered to be the work of the devil. All medical schools and universities excluded women, except for the Italian medical school at Salerno. It is thought to have been headed by a woman, Trotula (Dam Trot), in C.E. 1050. She was a foremost authority on medicine, and her work was quoted for centuries. In the 15th and 16th centuries, witch-hunting was used as a political cleansing of grassroots herbal practice to protect the growth of the professional medical guilds.

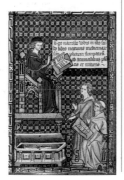

RIGHT *The Arab physician Avicenna left records of more than 800 herbs in the* Qanun.

THE PHYSICIANS OF THE MYDDVAI

This family of Welsh herbalists, with its roots in the Druidic tradition, flourished from the 10th century onward. In the 12th century they started a written record and history of their herbs and healing methods, called *The Physicians of Myddvai*. Traces of their tradition can still be found in Wales.

PARACELSUS (1493–1541)

Born Philippus Theophrastus Bombastus von Hohenheim, Paracelsus was a Swiss physician and alchemist who, like Nicholas Culpeper a century or so later, taught and wrote in his native tongue. Contemptuous of the quacks of the time, he postulated a simple form of herbalism based on his observation and experience of folk medicine. Believing that plants (and metals) contained different active ingredients, he pioneered the use of specific treatment for particular diseases.

THE RENAISSANCE

This was the Golden Age of Herbals. During the 16th century the world was expanding and plants from the newly discovered countries, such as yucca and nasturtium, stimulated interest and enquiry. Medical knowledge began to increase and many renowned herbals were published. Accurate observation and classification of plants are reflected in some of these beautiful books, notably those by Elizabeth Blackwell, John Gerard, John Parkinson, William Turner, and William Coles.

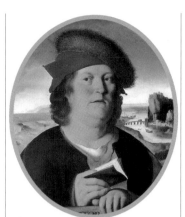

ABOVE *Paracelsus revolutionized Western medicine with his theories of herbal medicine.*

NICHOLAS CULPEPER (1616–54)

The astrologer and physician Nicholas Culpeper believed that everyone, including the common people, had a right to good and vibrant health, and so he translated the *London Dispensary* from Latin (a language only understood by the rich and educated) into common English, allowing ordinary people to read the work. In so doing, he upset the elitist academics of the time. He angered other physicians by writing *The English Physician*, "whereby a man may preserve his body in health; or cure himself, being sick, for three pence charge." He further enraged the apothecaries by suggesting that local plants were as good, sometimes better, than expensive imports. His book, *The Pharmacopoeia of Herbal Medicine*, usually known as *Culpeper's Herbal*, gives precise information on how to find and prepare plants for medicinal use, as well as suggesting which herbs to use for a particular complaint. It has remained in continuous print ever since it was first published.

SAMUEL THOMPSON (1769–1843) AND DR. COFFIN (1790–1866)

Samuel Thompson learned the Native American use of plants and healing traditions as a child. He developed a system of botanical medicine and wrote a series of handbooks. By the late 1830's he had millions of followers, but the popularity of botanicals worried the chemical practitioners, and jealous feuds developed. Dr. Coffin, a follower of Thompson's work, became disheartened, packed up his medicines, and left for Europe. He settled in the north of England, where he set up in practice and founded schools. With the plants that he had brought with him, Dr. Coffin was able to add a number of Native American plants to the European pharmocopoeia. In 1864, he helped set up the National Association of Medical Herbalists, now the National Institute of Medical Herbalists (N.I.M.H.).

FLOWER REMEDIES

Flower remedies, are made specifically to harness the effect that flowers have on the mood and vital spirit. Dr. Edward Bach began isolating these effects into remedies in England early in the 20th century. In Australia, wild flowers are made into Bush remedies for similar reasons. Flower remedies are easy to buy, make, and use.

How Herbalism Works

We know that herbs work medicinally because they have been tested by humans for thousands of years. During this time useless or harmful practices were discontinued,

LEFT *A herb may be classified as any plant used medicinally.*

psychotropic herbs were singled out and reserved for religious purposes, and what endured were the most useful medicinal herbs.

WHAT IS A HERB?

For the purposes of this book a herb is any plant used in medicine. Anything of a vegetative nature, that is used to make a remedy, may be called a herb, whether it is the flowers (camomile, elderflower, marigold), bark (willow), leaf (sage, rosemary, comfrey), stem (angelica), bulbs (garlic, onion), seeds (fennel), gel (aloe), or root (elecampane, mallow, dandelion). Lichens (Iceland moss), seaweed (bladderwrack), and fungi (Ganoderma) are also used.

HOW HERBS WORK

Herbs are very complex organisms, which when analyzed by such methods as gas chromatography are found to contain dozens of constituents that might be used to make medicines. A pharmacologist would isolate the active ingredient, but a herbalist believes that "nature knows best" and that the many compounds present in herbs are more effective when working together. It is inaccurate to extrapolate from laboratory studies, to say "x does this." It may act this way on its own, but its effects will change when it is accompanied by other ingredients and taken

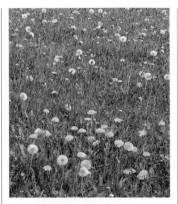

ABOVE *According to the herbal tradition, herbs such as the dandelion, work best when all their compounds are utilized.*

internally. The complex action may be direct – for example, an astringent or an irritant laxative – or subtle, such as the water-balancing qualities of dandelion. It may involve strategies unknown to present-day science.

Although research has shown the value of the traditional use of whole herbs, we know very little about the way herbs act within the human body. Modern science is poorly suited to the task: much medical knowledge comes from pathology (the study of the effects of disease as seen by dissection of a dead body) and by research on animals. This knowledge has little relevance to the

study of whole-plant remedies in the living body and to the holistic practice of medicine. A new methodology is needed. The N.I.M.H. together with many other professional groups of natural therapists are looking at this problem. Computer imaging and life modeling, the electron microscope, and computer-assisted tomography (C.A.T.) scans offer exciting new possibilities.

Herbal medicine occupies the middle ground between drugs and foods. At one end of the herbal spectrum are powerful plants, some of which have been used as the source of modern drugs, such as atropine from deadly nightshade. At the other end are nourishing plants such as nettle, rich in iron, vitamins, and amino acids.

Herbs have no side effects in the orthodox way. There may be indications and contraindications, but all effects are the result of the plant's character and the therapeutic strategy. There are no wanted or unwanted constituents: the whole plant is accepted just as it is. For example, sage has relaxing, stimulant, carminative, diuretic, diaphoretic, hormone-balancing, and febrifugal actions. All these are

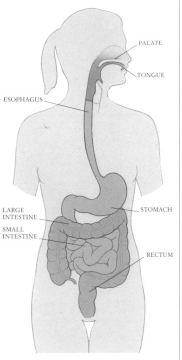

PALATE

TONGUE

ESOPHAGUS

LARGE INTESTINE

SMALL INTESTINE

STOMACH

RECTUM

ABOVE *The chemical make-up of plants is extremely complex and we still have little understanding on how they act on the body's system.*

part of its individual character and must be accepted, even celebrated, when it is taken.

With the growth of allopathic medicine and the development of the synthetic drug industry in the 20th century, the direct use of these plants in medicine became unpopular for a time in the Western world; old stories about such remedies sounded quaint and the rationale uncomfortable to the modern mind. It is only relatively recently that we have become more open-minded about herbalism as a system of medicine.

THE CONSTITUENTS OF ASPIRIN AND SAGE OIL

The one constituent of aspirin makes it easy to study and synthesize. Its effects are predictable. Although 100 percent effective in the laboratory, it will only be 75 percent effective in real life, because it may be taken inappropriately, for the wrong condition, in the wrong amount, or by a person with a constitution that can overcome its effects.

Essential oils are quite well researched yet they are only one percent of a plant's constituents. The whole plant is much more complex. A list may look comprehensive but many constituents have merely been identified and named and their precise action remains a mystery.

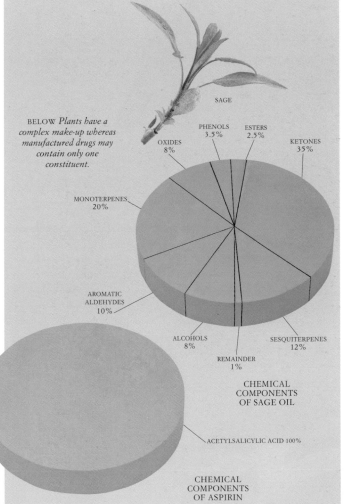

SAGE

BELOW *Plants have a complex make-up whereas manufactured drugs may contain only one constituent.*

PHENOLS 3.5%

ESTERS 2.5%

KETONES 35%

OXIDES 8%

MONOTERPENES 20%

AROMATIC ALDEHYDES 10%

ALCOHOLS 8%

SESQUITERPENES 12%

REMAINDER 1%

CHEMICAL COMPONENTS OF SAGE OIL

ACETYLSALICYLIC ACID 100%

CHEMICAL COMPONENTS OF ASPIRIN

The Chemical Components of Herbs

THERE IS MUCH *to be learned from pharmacologists but the further insight that can be gained from studying the chemistry of herbs should widen understanding and knowledge of herbalism – not reduce it. Herbs should never be taken because of the action of one particular chemical but instead for the combined action of the many chemical components that are found in a single plant.*

ABOVE *Yarrow has excellent diuretic properties.*

No herb should be taken only because it contains a certain constituent. This can lead to misleading and inaccurate practice as the constituent may be irrelevant in the overall mixture. It may be buffered, enhanced, or suppressed by other substances in the plant, or they could all work together in synergetic harmony.

ALKALOIDS

A chemical rather than a pharmacological grouping and the actions of its members are variable. They are often the most active constituents; indeed many modern drugs are derived from plant alkaloids, including morphine, caffeine, and nicotine. In the plant vervain, the alkaloids contribute to the relaxing quality of the herb.

BELOW *Some plants, such as rhubarb, have laxative properties.*

ANTHRAQUINONES

These are laxative. Herbs in this group include senna, rhubarb root, aloes, and yellow dock.

CYANOGENIC GLYCOSIDES

These are used to soothe the heart and lungs as they are sedating. They can be found in hawthorn.

FLAVONOIDS

Flavonoids strengthen blood vessels, improve peripheral circulation, and are anti-inflammatory. They are found in remedies for high blood pressure, failing circulation, and varicose veins. Some are diaphoretic or diuretic, improving circulation to the skin and kidneys respectively. These properties can be found in citrus fruits, buckwheat, yarrow, hawthorn, St. John's wort, gingko, and many other herbs.

RIGHT *For dry, unproductive coughs, try remedies that have a demulcent quality; for example, a carob drink.*

MUCILAGE AND GUMS

These have a demulcent (soothing, relaxing, and cooling) action. They are used in remedies for dry and unproductive coughs, inflamed and irritable stomach and bowels (soothing the gut), and inflamed bladders. Good sources are marshmallow root or leaf, linseed, and carob drinks.

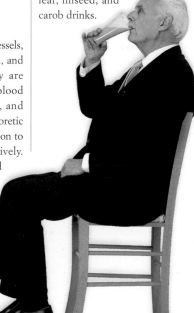

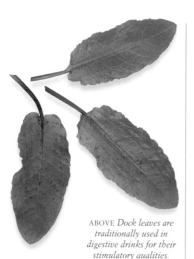

ABOVE *Dock leaves are traditionally used in digestive drinks for their stimulatory qualities.*

RESINS

Resins are sticky, oil-soluble substances usually including a volatile oil. It is thought that resins are secreted by plants as a protection against infection. Resinous plants used for their healing action include marigold and sage. These herbs are very useful in mouthwashes and gargles, since they are not easily washed away.

SALICYLATES

Salicylates are chemicals related to aspirin. They are analgesic, antiseptic, and anti-inflammatory. These chemicals are found in many herbal remedies for arthritis, including meadowsweet and willow bark. Unlike aspirin, herbal remedies that contain salicylates do not irritate the stomach, because they contain other constituents that protect the stomach lining – a good example of synergy in action.

RASPBERRY LEAF

SAPONINS

Saponins are named after their soap-like (emulsifying) action. This cleansing and softening property makes herbs that contain saponins useful for treating skin problems, both internally and externally. Chickweed and oats are good examples. Some saponin-rich plants have a hormone-like effect on the body. Examples include wild yam, which was used in the manufacture of the contraceptive pill.

TANNINS

Tannins are anti-inflammatory, antiseptic, and styptic. They are responsible for the astringency of herbal remedies. Strong tea owes its puckering taste to tannin. They can be found in many herbal remedies for wounds – for example, raspberry and horsetail.

VOLATILE OILS

Also known as essential oils, these are probably the best known of all plant constituents. These are the oils that are extracted from plants and used in aromatherapy. They are in themselves complex mixtures of constituents. Most herbs containing essential oils are antiseptic, antifungal, and work to stimulate the immune system. Thyme, marigold, and lavender are good examples of this. Many herb oils have anti-inflammatory properties, such as camomile. Ginger is an example of an essential oil used for its warming, carminative, and relaxing actions, both improving the circulation and relaxing spasm.

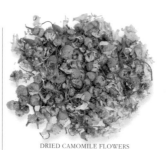

DRIED CAMOMILE FLOWERS

BITTER PRINCIPLES

This is a herbalist's rather than a pharmacologist's classification. The bitter taste of many herbal remedies is due to a variety of constituents, which are an important group for the herbalist. Bitter herbs stimulate the digestion, improve absorption of nutrients, normalize peristalsis, and improve liver function. This is why bitter herbs such as dandelion, dock, and marigold are an important and vital ingredient in many traditional digestive drinks.

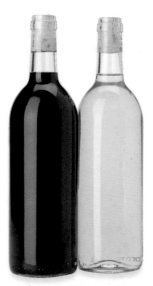

ABOVE *Many digestive drinks contain bitter herbs, which stimulate the digestive system and aid nutrient absorption.*

19

Gathering Herbs

GREEN PLANTS *are all around us, even in the inner city. In an emergency the dandelion that grows in a town or city can be gathered and used (but not if it is close to the dust and pollution from traffic). There are three ways to obtain good-quality, unadulterated, and accurately identified herbs: grow your own, pick them from the wild, or buy them from a retail supplier.*

GROWING YOUR OWN HERBS

Any small sunny space, even a windowsill, can be used to grow herbs. The major herbs, used in both cooking and medicine, are easy to grow. Some, like the mints, are so enthusiastic that they may have to be constrained in a pot. The rules of growing are simple: prepare the soil to the plant's liking and buy good-quality seeds from a reputable seller. There are many who run excellent mail order services. Order them by their Latin name, since many plants, such as sage and thyme, have many decorative garden varieties and the choice can be confusing. All varieties can be used to some extent, but the best for medicinal use have the species name *officinale* or *officinalis*. Seeds bought for gardening purposes, such as fennel or celery, have usually been sprayed and should never be used to make a herbal medicine.

It is a joy to watch plants growing, changing through the seasons, and preparing to flower. It is a pleasure to tend them, knowing that they will tend the whole family in due season. Some people talk to their plants, and it is easy to understand why. Home-grown herbs that are happy and healthy make excellent remedies.

Some plants are poisonous and should not be grown within the reach of young children. Children find it difficult to differentiate between harmful and non-harmful plants, especially if they have been taken blackberrying and know plants are orally gratifying and a major source of nourishment. Avoid growing plants with poisonous fruits and berries such as laburnum (*Laburnum anagyroides*), yew (*Taxus baccata*), lily-of-the-valley (*Convallaria majalis*), box (*Buxus sempervirens*), and holly berries (*Ilex aquifolium*).

BELOW Herbs are extremely easy to cultivate. Most herbs will grow happily in small pots on your windowsill.

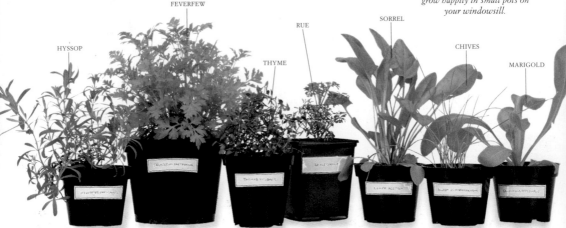

HYSSOP · FEVERFEW · THYME · RUE · SORREL · CHIVES · MARIGOLD

HARVESTING AND DRYING HERBS

Plants wilt quickly and the sooner they are prepared for use after picking the better.

LEAVES

Gather on a dry day. If you want only the young leaves of nettle, for example, these are best in spring when the plant has fresh energy, or in late summer when the plant is having a second growth spurt. When collecting leaves and stems (motherwort, burdock, dock), pick just before the plant comes into flower. Leaves collected for their aroma (rosemary, sage, lemon balm) are best gathered at midday, when their oil content is highest. To dry, tie into loose bunches and hang in a warm dry place. Leaves for poultices – for example, comfrey and plantain – can be collected to use fresh when needed, at any time of day and in any weather conditions.

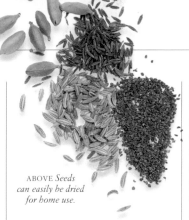

ABOVE *Seeds can easily be dried for home use.*

FLOWERS

Pick in the morning, after the dew has dried but before the flowers have become dehydrated by the hot sun. To dry, tie in loose bunches, or lay out on cloth or plain paper. (Do not use printed paper as the finish and ink will contaminate the herb.) Flowers are delicate so avoid direct sunlight or artificial heat.

SEEDS

Pick in the late afternoon or early evening when the plant is as dry as possible. Pick the whole stem, tie a paper bag over the seed heads, and hang upside down until completely dry. The seeds will then be easy to shake loose and collect in the bottom of the bag.

ROOTS

For reasons of conservation, roots should never be collected from the wild but only from your own garden sources. Roots are most potent in the fall, when they contain the plant's winter store. The roots of some perennials, such as echinacea and elecampane, can be harvested when the plant is being divided, while others, such as dandelion, which has one long tap root, will need to be resown for the next gathering season.

To harvest, carefully dig up the entire root and shake off any loose soil. You can then wash the root gently in cold running water and pat dry, but this is not always necessary. Dry in a warm place with a good air flow. Check and turn the root daily. When it is completely dry, remove any remaining soil with a soft brush. Do not peel the root as this will cause many of the important ingredients to be lost. For the same reason, do not cut the root until you are just about to use it.

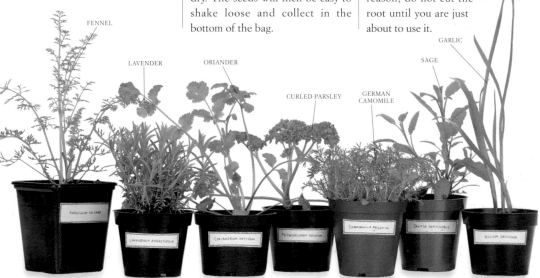

FENNEL

LAVENDER

ORIANDER

CURLED PARSLEY

GERMAN CAMOMILE

SAGE

GARLIC

PICKING YOUR OWN HERBS FROM THE WILD

Sometimes called wild crafting, gathering armfuls of herbs from a wild area was once a common activity, but today it is much more difficult. Many areas have been sprayed with chemicals and it is frequently illegal to pick plants from wild places. All habitats, even in remote areas, are under pressure from human activities and the need for conservation dictates that picking be limited.

Herbalists are worried that some plants may become extinct through thoughtless gathering. Herbalists in the U.S. voluntarily limit the collection of echinacea, golden seal, and lady's slipper to allow the wild stock to recover. The call for herbs is immense and ever growing as herbal remedies become validated by science and demanded by patients. The wild habitat cannot meet the demand and plants such as echinacea, and even St. John's wort, need to be cultivated. Commercial cultivation is in its infancy but it is developing and many herbs are now available from small, organic growers. Wild herbs will still need protection, however, to insure biodiversity.

Different countries have many different rules on conservation, so it is important to find out what the rules are before you pick plants, and to

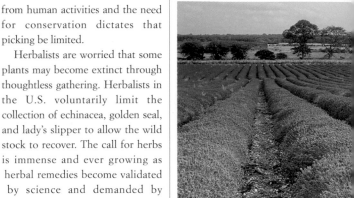

LEFT *Gather your herbs responsibly from wild habitats. Only pick what you really need and leave enough for new growth.*

know that you have permission to pick. Take with you a good well-illustrated guide to plants so that you can identify the plants accurately. Pick thoughtfully and take only the minimum you need. Gather away from roadsides, dogs, pollution, and spraying. Pick from healthy plants, taking a small amount from each plant and leaving enough for regeneration.

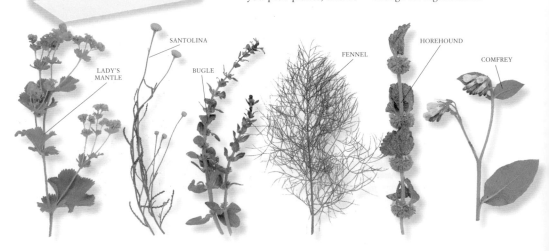

LADY'S MANTLE

SANTOLINA

BUGLE

FENNEL

HOREHOUND

COMFREY

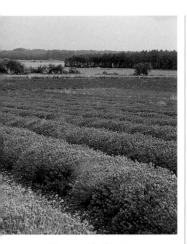

ABOVE *Commercial cultivation is becoming more common as consumer demand for herbal products grows.*

ACCURATE IDENTIFICATION

Many plants look extremely similar and can only be identified accurately when in flower or seed. Some members of the *Umbelliferae* family are toxic, so it is best to avoid these unless you are absolutely certain about identification.

If possible try to pick only common plants that you know well.

Dandelion, meadowsweet, comfrey, burdock, linden, and dock are all easy to identify.

Buy a good plant key and join a class to study the subject. This will involve going on expertly guided identification walks.

BUYING HERBS

You can buy dried herbs; both leaves and roots, from specialty shops and healthfood stores. Common names can cause confusion so always ask for what you want by its specific Latin name.

The popularity of natural remedies has generated a huge growth in the range and complexity of herbal products. Cosmetics are enhanced with herbal extracts of variable quality, while some manufacturers are working hard to produce safe and standardized therapeutics. The law protects us from grandiose and illegal claims but, as in all consumer transactions, it is for the buyer to beware. To avoid the huge cost involved in registering a product for human medical use, many herbs are sold as

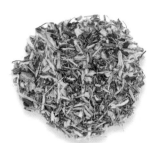

ABOVE *Many specialty shops and healthfood stores now sell dried herbs.*

supplements rather than medicines, but they must still be treated with respect. Many products still follow traditional formulas but single-herb tablets and capsules are increasingly available. For example, ginkgo, feverfew, and echinacea may all be bought in single form.

When buying, make sure that the product contains the herb that you need in a therapeutic amount. A reputable company will have done checks on the authenticity and purity of its herbal ingredients allowing you to purchase with confidence. Follow the dosage and pay careful attention to any cautions and contraindications.

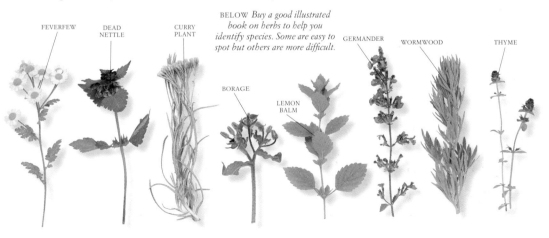

BELOW *Buy a good illustrated book on herbs to help you identify species. Some are easy to spot but others are more difficult.*

FEVERFEW   DEAD NETTLE   CURRY PLANT   BORAGE   LEMON BALM   GERMANDER   WORMWOOD   THYME

Making Herbal Preparations

There are many reasons, both practical and philosophical, for making your own herbal remedies. You can be sure that you are using ingredients only of the best quality and purity. Price too, is a factor – homemade remedies cost a fraction of the bought equivalent. And it is fun – children love making their own remedies. Wandering beside the hedgerows collecting rose hips or blackberries is health-giving in itself.

GENERAL RULES

For all preparations, assemble all the utensils and ingredients you need before you start.

Absolute cleanliness

Sterilize glass and metal by boiling in water for 20 minutes or placing in a medium oven for 20 minutes. Alternatively, use a proprietary sterilizing liquid. Caps and lids must also be clean. If a lid contains a small paper washer, remove it if it cannot be cleaned. When buying wholesale, bottles and lids are sold separately. Often there is a choice of several types of lid. If you are intending to recycle them, buy suitable lids to start with, and order extra paper inserts, or extra lids, in order to make up for wastage.

Follow the recipe

Doubling the amount of herbs that are used does not strengthen any mixture and it may even hinder the extraction processes.

Label fully and accurately

Give the name of the herb or preparation, together with the date. Adding the method of use and dosage to the label will also provide extra useful information.

Store appropriately

Use dark or amber glass, not plastic. Store safely, away from small children and animals.

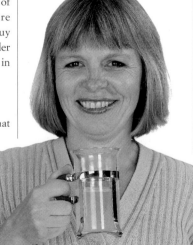

BELOW *When drinking teas, take time to inhale the aroma and feel the therapeutic effects throughout the body.*

WATER-BASED EXTRACTION

Using water is the simplest way to extract the active ingredients of herbs. Water-based remedies are also easy to drink and tolerate, even for children and those with a delicate constitution.

INFUSIONS (TEAS)

Some teas make refreshing and pleasant alternatives to Indian or China tea. Others, particularly decoctions, are an acquired taste.

✿ Method

1 tsp (5ml) of herbs per cup boiling water or ½ cup (1oz) dried or ¼–1 cup (1½–2oz/30g–45g) fresh herbs to 2½ cups (600ml) boiling water. Use pure boiled water, pour over the herbs, stir, put on a tight-fitting lid, and leave to brew as necessary.

• FLOWERS – camomile, linden, marigold – brew for 3 minutes.
• LEAVES – rosemary, thyme, parsley, etc. – brew for 3–5 minutes.
• HARD LEAVES, SEEDS, AND ROOTS – fennel seed, clove, elecampane root – brew 5–8 minutes.
• Strain, pour, and drink.

Herbal teas are drunk plain, without milk or sugar. Honey may be added if deemed essential.

As you drink the tea, remember the character of the herb and why you are taking it. Give the herb space and time to work.

Dosage

Standard adult dose: 1 cup three times a day. For acute conditions take 1 cup six times a day for one to three days until the condition improves. As a preventive or tonic, 1 cup twice a day is usually enough. In chronic conditions it may be necessary to take a tea for some months, although its effect should be noticeable within three to six weeks.

Doses for children

Give remedies proportionally. For example, for children over 15 years of age: give the adult dose, for children age 7 to 8: half adult dose; infants: 1 teaspoon only.

Infusions at the above strength may also be used as lotions and for compresses.

DECOCTIONS

A decoction involves simmering in water and is used to extract the properties of harder materials, such as roots, barks, and seeds and to make a stronger remedy than a tea.

The proportion of herb to water is the same as for tea.

Method

• ½ cup (1oz) dried or ¼–1 cup (1½–2oz/30–45g) fresh herbs to 2½ cups (600ml) water.
Chop or grind the herbs into small pieces. If the herbs are too hard to cut, soak them overnight in 2½ cups (600ml) water. Retain the water to use in the decoction and chop the softened herbs into pieces. Put the herbs and water into a pan, cover with a tight lid, and slowly bring to a boil. Once boiled, simmer gently for 10 minutes. Strain and add more water to make the liquid back up to 2½ cups (600ml).

Dosage

Standard adult dose: ½ cup two to three times day. Children proportionally (see Doses for children, above). A decoction will keep in the refrigerator for a few days.

REMEDIES FOR ANIMALS

It is not correct to assume that herbs are safe for animals just because they are natural remedies and can be used on humans. Animals have different metabolisms and different diseases to humans. It is best to obtain a diagnosis from your vet before attempting home treatment. Safe herbs for treating minor ailments in animals are: echinacea for infections and skin diseases of all kinds; camomile for irritability and stomach upsets; marigold for wounds, bites, and rashes.

Method
Use the dried herb to make 1 cup of the decoction or infusion, and reduce slowly over a low heat, to 2 tsp (10ml). Add an equal amount of brandy, shake well, and bottle. This makes 4 tsp (20ml), which will keep indefinitely.

Dosage:
For kittens and cats 2–10 drops twice daily; for large dogs 30 drops twice daily.

SYRUPS

Syrups are particularly useful for coughs and for children's ailments.

Method

To make a syrup, prepare a decoction as instructed. Return to the heat, remove the lid, and slowly reduce to 1½ cups (300ml). Then add 2 cups (1lb/454g) brown cane sugar or honey. Stir over the heat till the sugar has melted and the mixture is smooth and blended, taking care not to boil or burn. Pour into clean glass bottles. A syrup will last for several months.

Dosage

Adults: 2 tsp (10ml) three to six times a day. Children: 1 tsp (5ml) three to four times day.

Thyme cough syrup, (see p. 94).

CREAMS

Creams are an emulsion of oil and water, used to nourish and heal. They are lighter and cooler than ointments.

Powdered, tinctured, or decocted herbs, essential and infused oil can be added to any good quality, unscented skin cream.

Method

To 2 tbsp (30ml) base cream add ONE of the following. Blend in drop by drop until amalgamated.
• 5–15 drops essential oil
• 1–2 tsp (5–10ml) infused oil
• 1–2 tsp (5–10ml) strong decoction or tincture.
• 1–3 flat tsp (5–15ml) finely powdered herb.
• ½–1 flat tsp (2–5ml) powdered spice.

Alcohol-based Extraction

ALCOHOL HAS AN ACTIVE *and warming quality, and may be used to extract and preserve the active properties of a herb. It is a convenient way of storing remedies and so is becoming a major form of extraction for more and more herbs, not always appropriately. Alcohol is an appetizer and enhances the properties of digestive herbs, whereas water is better for sweet, cooling, or demulcent herbs. Alcohol of various strengths is used to extract different herb constituents. Resins need a strong alcohol, whereas tannins and some aromatic principles may be extracted in vinegar or a light beer. The alcohol strength given below is suitable for general home use.*

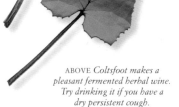

ABOVE *Coltsfoot makes a pleasant fermented herbal wine. Try drinking it if you have a dry persistent cough.*

Alcohol may be poorly tolerated by some people, produce allergies, or be unsuitable for religious reasons. Always check.

It is easy to forget that a tincture taken as a medicine, or a medicinal wine taken as a delicious aperitif, contains alcohol. Tinctures are similar in strength to spirits and should be counted as such when deciding on a safe driving limit.

TINCTURES

Tinctures are antiseptic and can be used internally and externally, in gargles, douches, compresses, liniments, washes, and baths.

Method

3½ cups (7oz/200g) dried herbs or 7 cups (14oz/400g) fresh herbs
4½ cups (1 liter) of liquid made up of three parts vodka to two parts water.

Put herbs in a large clean amber jar and pour the liquid over. Seal and store in a cool dark place for two weeks, shaking occasionally. Strain through a cloth and wring out all the liquid. Bottle, and label with name and date.

Dosage

Standard adult dose: 1 tsp (5ml) three times a day for chronic conditions;
1 tsp (5ml) six times a day for acute conditions (unless otherwise stated).

HERBAL WINES

Recipes for enjoyable fermented herbal wines such as elderflower or coltsfoot wine, will be found in many wine-making books. The recipes here are for infused wines, which are made by steeping herbs and spices in a good-quality wine.

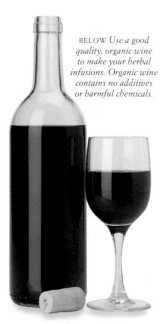

BELOW *Use a good quality, organic wine to make your herbal infusions. Organic wine contains no additives or harmful chemicals.*

Digestives, tonics, and aperitifs can all be made this way.

Since many people are allergic to wine, to the additives, or to the chemicals used to produce it, make sure you use a good-quality wine, preferably organic.

Nettle Beer

- 1lb (450g) malt extract
- 1 cup (6oz/175g) brown sugar
- 2¼lb (1kg) nettle tops
- 7 pints (4 liters) water
- ½oz (15g) yeast

Method

☞ Dissolve malt and brown sugar in warm water. Rinse nettle tops and then boil in 4 pints (2.3 liters) water for 30 minutes. Cool, strain, liquid into a clean bucket, top up with water to 4 pints (2.3 liters), add yeast, and leave to ferment for 5–6 days.

☞ When fermented and settled, pour into 8 bottles (leaving an air space of 2in [5cm]). Stopper very tightly and leave for two weeks. Serve cool.

Christopher's Digestive Tonic Wine and Winter Warmer

- 1 bottle wine
- 2-in (5-cm) piece fresh ginger root, grated
- 1 cinnamon stick
- 8 cardamom pods, crushed
  Sprig of rosemary
  Pinch allspice [optional]

Dosage

☞ A small wine glass 2 tbsp (1oz/30ml) daily as a warming tonic, or 1 tsp (1oz/15ml) in warm water to prevent chills.

Method

☞ Open the bottle and pour out a small amount. Add the other ingredients and recork. Stand for two weeks, shaking occasionally. Strain and rebottle.

ALLSPICE

ROSEMARY

GINGER

CARDAMOM

CINNAMON

RIGHT *The ingredients used to make Christopher's Digestive Tonic Wine and Winter Warmer.*

HERBAL BEERS

Beer is nutritious and cooling on a hot day. There are many traditional recipes, such as nettle beer (*see above*), in books on brewing.

MEDICINAL VINEGARS

Vinegar is a mild acid and is used as a preservative. Internally, it is cooling, cleansing, and slightly diuretic. Externally, it is antiseptic and cooling.

Thyme vinegar

This vinegar is a useful remedy as a general antiseptic. Drink for sore throats, gum disease, and coughs.

✿ Method

Loosely fill a jar with dried or fresh thyme. Cover with cider vinegar. Stand in a cool dark place, shaking occasionally. After two weeks strain, bottle the vinegar, and label.

✿ Dosage

Dilute one part vinegar with three parts water and use as a lotion for fungal and yeast infections such as athlete's foot and thrush. To use as a douche, dilute with ten parts water.

Fall fruit vinegar

This ruby red vinegar is an excellent remedy for soothing coughs, cutting phlegm, and cooling children's fevers. Blackberries or raspberries are traditionally used in this recipe.

✿ Method

Fill a jar with the washed fruit. Cover the fruit completely with cider or wine vinegar. Strain off after two weeks.

✿ Dosage

1–2 tsp (5–10ml) in water to taste, each morning for sluggishness and as a cleanser.
1 tsp (5ml) in water (honey may be added) for coughs and mild fevers. Drink freely.

Infused Oils

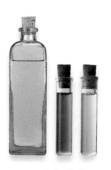

INFUSED OILS CAN BE USED *as rubs, massage oils, chest rubs, and liminents, or thickened with beeswax to make an ointment or salve. Herbal oils are soothing and lubricating. Some, such as almond oil and coconut oil, can nourish the skin, while others such as petroleum jelly make a protective barrier and retain heat. For herbal infusions a light oil, such as sunflower or grapeseed, is preferable to olive oil, which may overwhelm the natural fragrance of herbs. Traditionally, animal fats (lard and suet) were used.*

ABOVE *Infused oils can be used in a variety of ways, including ointments.*

The following methods of infusion can be used with oil of any origin. Leaves and roots are infused twice, spices and seeds once. Delicate flowers are best infused naturally in sunshine.

INFUSED HERB OIL FOR LEAVES, ROOTS, AND STEMS

Suitable herbs include comfrey, sage, rosemary, thyme, birch leaves, and elecampane.
You will need:
• Fresh or dried herbs.1½ cup (2oz/ 60g) fresh herb or ½ cup (1oz/30g) dried herb to 2½ cups (600ml) oil or jelly.
• Pure unblended vegetable oil, or petroleum jelly.
• Water bath, bain-marie, or steamer.

ᵫ Method

Use a pan with a tight-fitting lid. Put half the herbs loosely into the pan and cover completely with oil. Place the pan in a water bath, bain-marie, or steamer and simmer gently for 2 hours. Do not use direct heat or the

oil may burn and spoil. After 2 hours strain well and discard the spent herbs. The oil will have changed color, and absorbed some of the qualities of the herbs.

Repeat this process with the remaining herbs, covering them with the strained oil from the first batch. Return to the water bath and simmer for 2 hours. Strain well again. The oil will now have a deep rich herbal color.

Decant into clean amber glass bottles, label, and date. If you used fresh plant material, there may be a water residue beneath the oil.

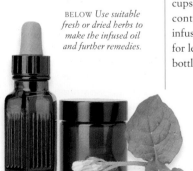

BELOW *Use suitable fresh or dried herbs to make the infused oil and further remedies.*

Discard this, as it will spoil the oil. The keeping properties of infused oil can be enhanced by the addition of 10 percent wheatgerm oil or vitamin E oil.

Infused oil for spices

Use powdered spices such as cayenne, mustard, fennel, pepper, and cloves. Spices are stronger than herbs and so far less is needed.

ᵫ Method

The exact amount of spice you use will depend on the size of the container. As an average, use ½ cup (2oz/60g) powdered spice to 2½ cups (600ml) vegetable oil. Fill the container with spices and oil and infuse in a water bath as described for leaves above, for 2 hours. Strain, bottle, and label.

CAUTION

Do not use "pepper" oils on broken skin or near eyes. Wash hands after use.

Infused oil for flowers

Flowers such as roses, linden, or St. John's wort are too delicate to infuse over direct heat; infusion by sunlight produces better results.

✵ Method

Put the flowers into a clean, clear glass jar. Cover with oil and leave to stand in direct sunlight for four weeks. St. John's wort oil will turn red when it is ready. You may need to strain some oils and add more petals to achieve a reasonable strength, repeating as necessary. Strain the finished oil into clean amber glass bottles, label, and date.

The following remedies can be made using infused oil.

Ointment

Use ointments to soothe and heal. They do not soak into the skin but they make a protective barrier. Comfrey ointment is a valued remedy. Its versatility is extended when it is warmed with 4 drops of rosemary or lavender essential oil. Use for all types of cuts, bruises, sprains, aches, pains, arthritic stiffness. Apply liberally.

✵ Method

2½ tbsp (40ml) infused herb oil
1 tsp (4g) beeswax
2–8 drops of essential oil (optional)
Grate or chop the beeswax and melt slowly into the oil over a water bath. Pour into a clean jar, label, and date.

Liniment

A medicated liquid containing oil and alcohol, liniment is applied to the skin to relieve pain or stiffness. An excellent all-purpose liniment comprises marigold and echinacea tincture with St. John's wort and bay leaf infused oil.

✵ Method

4 tbsp (60ml) infused herb oil
4 tbsp (60ml) tincture
5–10 drops essential oil (optional)
Mix together, bottle, and label. Shake well before use.

Lip salve

Make a soothing and protective winter lip salve from equal parts of camomile, marigold, and rose petals.

✵ Method

Infuse the herbs in a mixture of 3 parts cocoa butter to 1 part wheatgerm or almond oil in a water bath for 2 hours. Strain and pour into clear jars.

ESSENTIAL OR VOLATILE OILS

These volatile and aromatic principles of a plant (see p. 19) are extracted from their flowers (e.g., rose, jasmine), leaves (e.g., rosemary), or roots (e.g., ginger). Pure essential oils should not be used undiluted or taken internally. In nature they are found at concentrations of 5 percent or lower, and this is a suitable dilution to start with. They work much better at low dilutions. Use essential oils to make the following soothing and refreshing remedies.

Spray

Make a cooling wash, or room spray with 5 drops of essential oil to 2½ cups (600ml) water.

Massage oil

Five percent essential oil to a base vegetable oil makes a general purpose massage oil for tired or aching muscles.

Bath

Add 5–15 drops of one or more essential oils to a bath. Rosemary is ideal. Relax, breathe deeply to clear the head, improve circulation, and generate a refreshing feeling. Do not have the bathwater too hot or the bath will become enervating rather than invigorating.

Decongestant chest rub

Mix into 4 tsp (20ml) vegetable oil or petroleum jelly, 5 drops peppermint, 5 drops eucalyptus, 5 drops basil, and 5 drops thyme essential oils. Rub onto the chest and back at bedtime. The oil evaporates throughout the night, keeping the air passages clear.

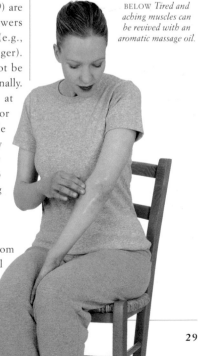

BELOW *Tired and aching muscles can be revived with an aromatic massage oil.*

Preparations

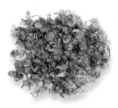

The most common way of using herbs to treat ailments at home is to use a single herb to respond to a particular condition. This is known as "simples." One herb may be used in a variety of different ways. For example, camomile tea is drunk for restless stress or a cold camomile compress can be applied to dry, itchy eyes. This flexibility makes it possible to use the right herb in the right way, with the minimum of intervention.

ABOVE *Camomile is an example of a herb that can be used as a simple.*

Using simples skillfully is one of the pleasures of herbal medicine. They may be used in a variety of ways.

Pastes

Pastes are used to draw foreign bodies or infections to the surface of the skin. Boils, splinters, and abscesses can all be treated in this way. Pastes can also be used to draw heat from swollen, inflamed, or sprained muscles or joints. All pastes have a base of holding material. This could be Iceland moss, slippery elm, mallow root, oats, fuller's earth, or betonite clay.

To make a healing and clearing paste for boils, mix 4 tsp (20ml) marigold tincture and

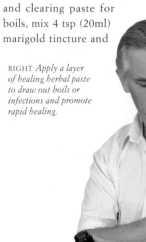

RIGHT *Apply a layer of healing herbal paste to draw out boils or infections and promote rapid healing.*

2 tsps (10ml) marshmallow root powder, adding water if necessary. Apply a thick layer to the skin, cover with plastic wrap, and then secure with a bandage. Renew the paste every four hours if necessary.

Poultices

Poultices are used to draw out infection, to soothe, warm, and promote elimination and healing. Take the fresh (or frozen) leaves of comfrey and blanch in boiling water to soften. Since the underside of the comfrey leaf is covered with hairs that can irritate the skin, either place the topside of the leaf on the skin or protect the skin first with a layer of light cheese-cloth. Build up two or three layers of leaf, cover with plastic wrap, and hold in place with a crepe bandage. Leave for 4 to 6 hours or overnight. Repeat dosage as needed.

Gargles

Gargling is an effective way of soothing the throat. It is also useful for gum problems, loose teeth, poor mouth tone, mouth sores, and thrush. Gargle frequently, four or more times daily. You can use any of the following as a gargle:
• TINCTURE one part tincture diluted with five parts water.
• TEA standard strength.
• DECOCTION 1:1 with water.
• VINEGAR 1:4 with water.
• A pinch of salt adds a soothing element, and a pinch of cayenne adds a stimulating antiseptic quality to all the above.
• Sage tea is specific for good mouth health and can be taken daily as a gargle or mouthwash.

Smoking mixtures

Sage, coltsfoot, and mullein are soothing plants with soft, furry leaves. They burn easily and the smoke is inhaled to soothe the chest. Aromatic herbs such as rosemary, lavender, thyme, fennel seed, and anise are added for their therapeutic effect and flavor. Tobacco (*see Coltsfoot, p. 97*).

Dry inhalant

Crush together equal parts of fennel seed, aniseed (not star), and thyme, and sprinkle on a burning charcoal block. Inhale the smoke for asthma, chest tightness, and wheeziness. Use nightly or when needed.

Smudge sticks

Used to fumigate people and homes, and can be bought or made. Their smoke helps to keep the air pure and the atmosphere clear.

Steam inhalants

Used therapeutically to clear the head and sinuses. Pour boiling water over aromatic herbs (e.g., sage, peppermint, lavender, rosemary, thyme) and inhale the steam. A few drops of essential oil will provide a stronger inhalant.

This can also be used as a squat, for delayed periods, painful periods, and cramps. Sit over the steam and simply relax.

Room sprays

Tea, a diluted tincture (one part tincture to 10 parts water), and a few drops of essential oil can be used in combination or singly to make a refreshing room spray. Use a light misting spray, of the type sold for spraying plants. A room spray will keep the air fresh, damp, and healthy, aid breathing, and reduce airborne bacteria.

A relaxing and disinfectant spray for a child with chesty cough:
• 1 cup camomile tea
• 3 drops eucalyptus oil
• 3 drops lavender oil
• Spray the room every four hours and at bedtime.

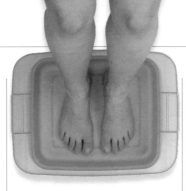

ABOVE *Warm hand and foot baths ease stiff and aching joints, and improve elimination and general circulation.*

Hand and foot baths

These can be the main part of a treatment and used every 6 hours, as part of a regular preventive regime, or used occasionally.

Teas are used at standard strength or diluted with an equal amount of water. Tinctures are diluted one part tincture to eight parts water. With essential oils, use 5 drops per pint of water.

If you suffer from stiff hands, use rosemary tea and a pinch of cayenne. The hand bath should be at blood temperature. Soak for 10–20 minutes.

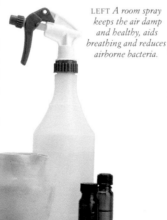

LEFT *A room spray keeps the air damp and healthy, aids breathing and reduces airborne bacteria.*

Mustard foot bath

1 tsp (5ml) mustard powder to 2½ cups (600ml) hot water is a valuable traditional remedy for circulation, and to prevent cold chills entering the bones.

Washes, compresses, and lotions

Herbal remedies can all be used directly on the skin as simple lotions, douches, compresses, and fomentation. Use any of the following:
• TEA at normal strength
• DECOCTION 1:1 with water
• TINCTURE 1:4 with water
• HERBAL VINEGAR diluted 1:6 with water

As a lotion, apply sparingly to the affected part and pat dry. Marigold tea makes an excellent lotion to clean and dress minor cuts, wounds, bites, and rashes.

A cool compress will soothe and draw out heat, inflammation, and irritation. Cool the liquid first in the refrigerator or by adding crushed ice. Soak a clean cloth or crepe bandage in the liquid and wrap it around the affected part. Cover to keep in place. Repeat every 2 hours if necessary. Camomile tea makes a cool, supportive compress for varicose veins. A hot compress will relieve cramps and muscle tension. Use rosemary or ginger.

Use hot and cold compresses alternately to stimulate circulation and draw abscesses.

Lotions (all except the vinegar dilution) can be used as an eye wash and compress for tired eyes. Dilute 1:1 with water and strain well. Always use freshly made lotions for the eyes and discard after use.

Materia Medica

ALL PLANTS HAVE AN *influence on the mood and emotions of humans. They speak directly to the vital spirit, helping to balance and promote physical and emotional well-being. Bear this in mind when choosing a specific herb for a person. Try to build a picture of each herb, bringing your objective and subjective skills together. Add practical understanding through the touch, taste, and smell of the herb. You can feel the softening qualities of*

ABOVE *Assess the mood of the patient to be treated before making a choice of herb for a particular complaint.*

coltsfoot leaf, taste the antiseptic qualities of thyme, and smell the warmth of angelica. Look at all the actions and all the uses; consider attributes such as hot or cold, soothing or stimulating, and in this way acquire an overall feeling for the herb and its therapeutic strategy. Each person responds to illness differently. When

LEFT *The value of herbs is that they address the whole body and help balance mind, body, and spirit.*

prescribing a remedy, it is important to know how illness affects the particular individual. Some people become angry that their body has "let them down"; they fight it and the illness, leaving little scope or time for healing. Others become depressed and lack the motivation to get well. Apathy makes it hard to focus on the vital spirit needed for healing. The patient's emotional state will affect their experience and influence the prognosis. Sometimes there is a choice between several diuretics or relaxants, and the choice will depend on the character and vital spirit of the person. A particular herb will not only be the best choice for a person's ailment, but also complement their character and mood. With practice these decisions will become intuitive.

RIGHT *Touch, taste, and smell the herbs that you use in your remedies to help build a complete profile.*

How to Use this Section

This section of the book contains profiles of 36 of the most commonly found herbs used to make remedies. In each case there is a general description of the herb and where to find it with a photographic illustration for identification. The detailed list of uses in the home, as well as professional and special uses, will guide you in your choices of herbal remedies. Information on the actions and character of each herb as well as its chemistry will add to your own knowledge of herbal medicine and the combination will provide a foundation for the skills of a herbalist.

All the herbs described are safe if used appropriately. Use the general knowledge you gain from this and other herb books, balanced and modified with the specific and expert knowledge you have of yourself and your family. Consider the herbs and plan a treatment, but if you are unsure in any way, do not proceed; seek professional advice if necessary.

BELOW **The 36 herbs illustrated in this section are each presented in a similar fashion for ease of reference.**

Principal uses in the home, together with recommended dosage and method of treatment.

Historical beliefs, myths, and practices concerning the plant.

Each herb section has a general description of the plant, detailing what it looks like and where it grows.

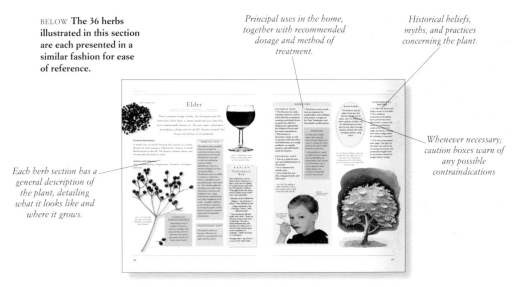

Whenever necessary; caution boxes warn of any possible contraindications

PROPERTIES OF HERBS

The properties of herbs cannot be described in narrowly defined terms. For example, while it is true to say that camomile is "good" for stressful headaches, this is not the whole truth. Aspirin may also be taken for a headache, but camomile and aspirin cannot be treated in the same way, nor can they be used as substitutes for each other. Aspirin has a specific action; camomile has more generalized effects. With camomile, the relief of the headache is just one of the benefits of the overall relaxing qualities of the herb. The light, open-faced camomile herb is warming (but not in the more stimulating way of ginger) with a bitter edge that reassures the liver, encouraging the process of digestion (mental and physical), soothing the frayed nerves, and thus easing mind and body.

The sufferer might need the clearing, sunshine warmth of marigold, the cool thoroughness of cleavers (*Galium aparine*), or the pungent, slightly aggressive fruit of the juniper.

Yarrow

ACHILLEA MILLEFOLIUM

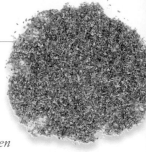

DRIED YARROW FLOWERS

Also known as milfoil, this healing plant has long been considered sacred in many cultures. Its old country names include nosebleed and carpenter's weed, allusions to its wound-healing properties. Yarrow is also without equal when it comes to reducing fevers.

General description

A beautiful, aromatic plant bearing flat heads of white or pink flowers in late summer at the top of straight, strong stems. It is found throughout the temperate regions of the world, either as a native or as a weed of cultivation. Yarrow prefers dry, grassy habitats but is a very adaptable survivor. The clusters of low-growing, feathery leaves are a familiar sight on lawns or pathways. In a meadow it opens out and becomes magnificent. Red-flowered cultivars have been developed for gardens, as it has a prolonged flowering season in the herbaceous border and even provides decoration when dried. The whole herb is used in herbalism.

ABOVE *The small white flattish flowers of the yarrow plant appear in the late summer.*

Actions and character

Styptic, antiseptic, astringent, anti-inflammatory, diaphoretic, carminative, antispasmodic, tonic for the venous system.

PROFESSIONAL USES

Hemorrhage – use large doses of an infusion of the fresh herb.
It is also used for nephritis, hypertension, and thrombosis, and as an adjunct in radiotherapy.

DOMESTIC USES

In the biodynamic system of gardening, yarrow tea is added to the compost heap to speed decomposition.
A few chopped leaves lend pungency to salads. The herb makes a pleasant and wholesome beer, and is used as a country cure for rheumatism.

BELOW *Yarrow stalks are traditionally thrown to read the I Ching, the ancient Chinese book of divination.*

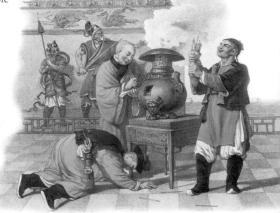

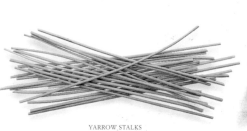

YARROW STALKS

HOME USE

INTERNAL USES
• Piles – internally and externally.
• To treat fevers, to induce sweating, and lower temperature; yarrow is suitable for childhood fevers.
• Poor circulation, cold feet, and problems from varicose veins.

• Period pains and pelvic pains from congestion, previous disease, and inflammatory conditions.

EXTERNAL USES
• As a cream or wash for inflamed wounds and weeping eczema.
• As a wound herb to stop bleeding and cuts that become inflamed.

HISTORICAL NOTES

❀ Yarrow's botanical name *Achillea* refers to the ancient Greek hero Achilles, who used it to cure spear wounds.

❀ A popular remedy for treating fevers and feverish conditions, yarrow was once used as a substitute for quinine.

❀ Native Americans burned yarrow to help drive away evil spirits.

❀ To understand the voice of yarrow, chew a little of the root and hold it in the mouth. A tea of leaf and flower will continue the story.

❀ Yarrow stalks are used when consulting the I Ching. The hexagrams are picked according to the way the stalks are thrown.

❀ European women used to throw it onto the fire and look into the flames for a picture of their future husband.

DOSAGE

May be taken freely in acute conditions. Drink three cups of tea daily for chronic conditions.

Tincture; 20 drops to 1 tsp (5ml) depending on circumstances.

A tea made with equal parts of elderflowers, peppermint, and yarrow is a pleasant drink and very effective for flu and other fevers. Drink the tea hot and frequently – up to a cup every 2 hours.

To relieve varicose veins quickly, add 30 drops of horse chestnut (Aesculus hippocastanum) tincture to a pint of yarrow tea and drink over a day. The same mixture can be used as a compress.

Use yarrow infused oil to treat varicose eczema conditions.

To stop bleeding, chew a few leaves (to soften and clean), and apply directly to the cut. (For the sake of hygiene chew your own leaves.)

Chew the fresh root for toothache.

Put yarrow in a bath or compress for painful joints.

CAUTION

The essential oil is contraindicated in pregnancy. Very large doses of fresh plant preparations are best avoided in early pregnancy.

CHEMICAL CONSTITUENTS

Essential oil including azulenes and eugenol, flavonoids, bitters, tannins.

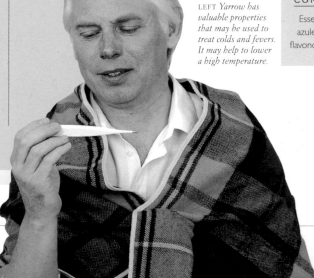

LEFT *Yarrow has valuable properties that may be used to treat colds and fevers. It may help to lower a high temperature.*

POWDERED GARLIC

Garlic

ALLIUM SATIVUM

*One of the most common kitchen herbs, garlic was originally
from central Asia but is now widely cultivated in most climates.
The garlic bulb consists of many individual cloves enclosed in a
white, papery skin. It has a strong odor and pungent taste.*

ABOVE *The garlic bulb
consists of many
separate cloves enclosed
by a purplish-white skin.*

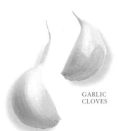

GARLIC
CLOVES

PROFESSIONAL USES

Garlic is used
professionally in the same
manner as in the home
and there are no
additional uses.

DOMESTIC USES

Even when used in
cooking, garlic still
benefits the circulation.
Garlic-infused oil
combined with cider
vinegar makes a good
salad dressing for people
with a weak digestion.

General description

An easily grown perennial plant with white, globular
flower-heads on a simple stem. It prefers a rich, sandy
soil. The underground bulb is used in herbal medicine.

Actions and character

Antiseptic, antiviral, fungicidal, antispasmodic,
expectorant, anti-allergic, lowers blood pressure, lowers
blood sugar and cholesterol, circulatory stimulant.

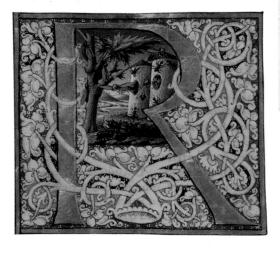

R E C I P E

Garlic Honey

This is a surprisingly pleasant
way of taking garlic, and well
tolerated by children. Both
garlic and honey are
antiseptic, making this
preparation an excellent
basic cure-all that should be
a standby in all households.
Use to prevent and treat
colds, infections,
and allergies.

• *2 whole heads garlic,
peeled and crushed*
• *1¼ cups (1lb/454g) honey*

☙ Put the garlic and a little of
the honey into a mortar and
pound together until the
garlic becomes completely
transparent. ☙ Add the rest
of the honey and mix well.
☙ Store in a clean jar.

Dosage: as a preventive, take
1 tsp (5ml) daily; as a
treatment for infections, take
3 tsp (15ml) daily. May also
be added to hot water and
lemon juice for sore throats
and colds, or to any other
herbal tea.

LEFT *Honey is a well-tried
and tested antiseptic remedy.
Mix with garlic for an
effective cough treatment.*

CHEMICAL
CONSTITUENTS

Volatile oil including the
sulphur compounds allicin
and alliin, B vitamins,
selenium, germanium,
flavonoids.

HOME USE

INTERNAL USES

• Garlic is an excellent long-term remedy for circulatory problems, helping to keep the arteries clear and strong and the blood pressure healthily low.
• Reduces the risk of circulatory problems in people with diabetes.
• Protects the heart.
• Disinfects and clears phlegm from the lungs; helps infected coughs, bronchitis, and asthma with sticky phlegm.
• Helps prevent colds, flu, and other viral infections. Relieves symptoms of sinusitis, hay fever, and excessive sneezing.
• Improves digestion of fats (taken with food).
• Kills intestinal worms.

EXTERNAL USES

• Infused oil for ear and nose infections (as drops).
• Infused oil as a chest rub (suitable for infants with coughs and colds).
• Pessary for vaginal and pelvic infections.
• Juice applied to warts and fungal infections including ringworm.
• Compress for abscesses.

DOSAGE

The odorous constituents of garlic are the source of its strength, and deodorized preparations do not work as well. To counteract the smell, take with fresh parsley.

Tablets of powdered garlic are the most useful type for long-term use. Enteric-coated tablets are available. These do not dissolve in the stomach and thus avoid regurgitation of the taste. Follow the recommendations on the package. Double the dose, for short periods, to ward off unpleasant colds and coughs.

For short-term use, to treat coughs, infections, and worms, take garlic honey or lightly roast a few cloves with their skin on and eat as many as you can.

For worms in children, simmer a clove or two in a cup of milk and give daily for three weeks.

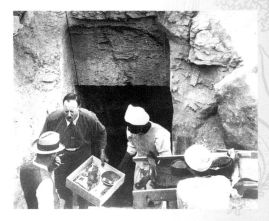

ABOVE *Garlic was known to the Ancient Egyptians. Cloves were found in the tomb of Tutankhamen in the Valley of the Kings.*

RELATED PLANTS

Onions, leeks, and wild garlic species share the same properties as garlic, but to a lesser extent. Onions are wetter, cooler, and more demulcent than garlic and more suitable for infants. Onion syrup can be made in the same way as garlic syrup. The dose for infants is 1–3 tsp (5–15ml) daily. Onion juice can be applied to infected spots and styes. In the Welsh herbal tradition, leek soup is recommended to combat "weakness caused by cold and damp weather."

HISTORICAL NOTES

Garlic has been used for many centuries as a strengthening and anti-infective food.

Nicholas Culpeper noted that it was called the poor man's cure-all by the ancients but wrote of its strong and offensive smell as unsuitable for people of a "choleric" or "melancholic" disposition.

European farm laborers said that eating garlic gave them the strength to work in the hot sun.

Cloves of garlic were found in the pharoah Tutankhamen's tomb.

CAUTION

Garlic can irritate the stomach, but its benefits are so great that it is worth finding a way to take it. Try the methods outlined under Dosage.

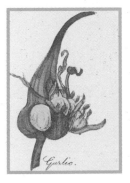

Garlic.

LEFT *Culpeper wrote about garlic's properties to "cure-all" complaints in his Herbal.*

Aloe

ALOE VERA

Aloe originates from Africa but is now grown in many countries and can be cultivated in temperate areas if protected from frost. It makes an excellent, unfussy house plant that should be grown in all kitchens, for instant use on burns.

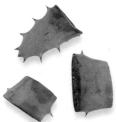

FRESH ALOE LEAVES

General description

Aloe or *Aloe vera* is a tropical member of the lily family with long, thick, succulent, dark green leaves with yellow-green streaks. The juice (gel) from the leaves is the part most used, fresh or preserved, but the whole leaf of this and other varieties is also used.

Actions and character

The gel promotes healing and is anti-inflammatory, antiseptic, and antifungal. Extracts of the whole leaves are strongly laxative and emmenagog. It also has cooling qualities.

LEFT *Originally from tropical Africa, aloe makes an attractive and useful house plant.*

LEFT *Aloe gel can be applied to burns or wounds for its antiseptic and cooling properties.*

CAUTION

Do not use internally in pregnancy as the anthraquinone glycosides are purgative. High doses of the leaves may cause vomiting.

PROFESSIONAL USES

Constipation and bowel disorders in cancer and immune deficiencies.

DOMESTIC USES

The aloe plant yields a deep purple dye.
The flower remedy is used as a restorative for people who are burned out and exhausted, especially from creative work of any kind.

CHEMICAL CONSTITUENTS

Mucilage, resin, anthraquinones, amino acids, and vitamins.

RUB DIRECTLY ONTO CUT

HOME USE

INTERNAL USES

• Use the transparent gel for burns, sunburn, radiation burns, insect bites, contact allergies from handling plants, dermatitis, eczema, inflamed and itchy skin conditions, leg ulcers, diaper rash, shingles, ulcers on the eye, dry and itchy scalps, ringworm, athlete's foot, mouth ulcers, and easing the pain of new dentures.

• Aloe gel, or a tincture of the gel, may be added to liniments for aches, pains, and swollen joints.

• Take internally for candidiasis, weak digestion, general weakness and anemia due to malabsorption, bloating, stomach ulcers, and gum disease.

• The yellow juice may be used as a laxative.

• Tea or tincture of the whole leaf is used internally for stubborn constipation, intestinal worms, and liver congestion.

EXTERNAL USES

• Apply the bitter yellow juice from the base of the leaves on fingernails to discourage nail biting.

• As a compress for painful, inflamed joints.

DOSAGE

The best preparation for the skin is the fresh gel. Simply cut a slice off the top of a leaf and squeeze the gel directly onto the skin. The cut end of the plant will seal over, allowing it to be used many times. Clumps of large aloe leaves can be bought in markets selling West Indian produce. They will keep for several months if stored in a cool place. Alternatively, the fresh leaves can be cut into healing patches and kept in the freezer.

Many preparations are now available in stores for both medicinal and cosmetic use.

The clear gel can be taken internally. Dosage: 1–2 tbsp (15–30ml).

As a laxative, use the whole leaf dried and powdered. Single dose: 100mg. Tincture dose: ½ –1½ tsp (2–8ml). For stubborn, chronic constipation take ½ tsp (2ml) twice daily. It is important to take a carminative herb, such as ginger or cinnamon, at the same time, to avoid griping. A few drops of ginger tincture will suffice. Compound pills are available.

FRESH ALOE HEALING PATCHES

Divide each aloe leaf in half lengthways, then cut into 2-in (5-cm) pieces. Wrap each piece in plastic wrap. Put loosely into a freezer bag so the patches do not stick together. Make at least 20. Label, date, and freeze. These leaves can be kept for six to nine months in the freezer.

To use as a lotion, unwrap and place the gel side against the skin and rub evenly over the affected area. It is not necessary to thaw. Repeat once or twice daily. To draw and cool, unwrap, place the gel side against the skin and hold the patch in place with a soft bandage. Repeat every 6 hours if needed.

HISTORICAL NOTES

❀ Aloe gel was known to the ancient Greeks and Romans as an excellent remedy for wounds, burns, and inflammatory diseases of the skin.

❀ In Muslim countries the plant is used as a symbol of patience.

❀ Aloes wood, as mentioned in the Bible, is from an entirely different plant (*Aquilaria agallocha*). It is from a tree grown in India and Malaysia for its aromatic properties and for use in incense.

BELOW *Aloe was known as a healing plant to the Ancient Greeks who used it to treat wounds.*

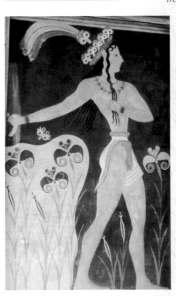

Marshmallow

ALTHEA OFFICINALIS

Marshmallow contains a healing mucilage and its Latin name
Althea comes from the Greek altho, meaning to cure.
Originally from China, marshmallow was used by the Ancient
Egyptians. It was formerly cultivated for its sweet-tasting roots,
which were traditionally used to make marshmallow confectionery.

DRIED
MARSHMALLOW
FLOWERS

MARSHMALLOW
FLOWER

General description

This beautiful perennial plant has pale pink, white, or
purple flowers and grows, as its name suggests, in
marshy places in temperate regions. The roots and
leaves are used in herbal medicine.

Actions and character

Demulcent, soothing, emollient,
nutritive. The classic
demulcent remedy.

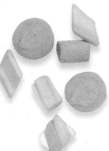

ABOVE *The marshmallow*
plant was the original
source of this popular
marshmallow candy.

LEFT *Marshmallow has*
attractive pink, purple,
or white tear-shaped
gray-green leaves.

CHEMICAL CONSTITUENTS

Mucilage, tannins,
flavonoids.

DOMESTIC USES

Mallow leaves may be
eaten as a vegetable,
cooked like spinach, or
chopped in salads. They
are traditionally eaten to
promote milk production
while breast-feeding.
Mallow and nettle leaves,
boiled with a little onion
and potato, make a
nourishing soup. The
flowers of any mallow
make a pleasing addition
to salads and a refreshing
herbal tea. The seeds have
a nutty taste and may be
eaten freely. The roots
make a palatable
vegetable if boiled and
then fried with onions.
The flower remedy is used
to develop openness and
trust in those who find it
hard to make friends.

PROFESSIONAL USES

Marshmallow is used in
the same manner as in the
home and there are no
current additional
professional uses.

RECIPE

Purple Cough Syrup

Children, especially, love the
color of this cough syrup.

• *3 handfuls of the deepest*
purple marshmallow flowers
• *2-in (5-cm) piece cinnamon*
stick (optional)
• *Sufficient honey to cover*

✿ Fill a jar with the flowers
and lightly press them down.
✿ Cover with honey and
leave to stand for two
weeks. ✿ Strain into clean
bottles, label, and store in a
cool place.

Dosage: 1 or 2 tsp (5 or
10ml) as needed, for dry and
irritable coughs and
loosening phlegm.

HOME USE

INTERNAL USES
• Mallow is soothing (demulcent) for any inflammation or irritation of the lungs, digestive system, and urinary tract.
• Bronchitis, dry coughs, mouth ulcers (as a mouth wash), sore throats, gastritis, peptic ulcers, hiatus hernia, enteritis, irritable bowel, dry constipation, kidney disease, kidney stones and gravel, cystitis.
• Dry skin, taken as an infusion for some months.
• Drink an infusion to redress dehydration after long air journeys.

EXTERNAL USES
• Use in poultices or creams to draw splinters, clean out wounds, and to resolve boils, abscesses, and ulcers.
• Apply in washes and compresses for weeping skin conditions.
• For insect bites and stings mix the powdered root with sufficient water to make a paste and apply. Fresh leaves may be rubbed directly onto stings and bites.

DOSAGE

May be taken freely whenever soothing is required. For maximum effect, soak 1oz (30g) of the root in 2½ cups (600ml) of cold water overnight and drink over the next day.

Marshmallow is not often used by itself but as an adjunct to other herbs. For example, use with thyme for coughs; with camomile and comfrey for hiatus hernia; with sage for painful breasts (internally and externally); with cleavers, thyme, or fennel for cystitis; and with cornsilk and dandelion leaf for kidney stones and water retention.

The powdered root makes an excellent base for poultices and hot fomentations as it holds the heat for a long time. To make a drawing cream for spots, add one part of powdered root to five parts of any good skin cream.

RELATED PLANTS

Many species and varieties of mallow grown as garden plants can be used as substitutes for marshmallow in medicine. These include the leaves and flowers of the garden hollyhock (Althea rosea), which originates from Asia, and the tree and bush mallows (Lavatera species) from southern Europe. Various wild mallows (Malva sylvestris and other species) are common weeds, and are also widely cultivated. Their flowers can be made into refreshing summer drinks.

HISTORICAL NOTES

Mallows have been used as food and medicine by many peoples. Mallow seeds are commonly used in Chinese medicine.

Marshmallow candies were originally made from the candied root, and used to soothe coughs. However, they no longer contain any mallow, only sugar, flour, and gum.

BELOW *The Chinese use the seeds of the mallow species in their traditional medicine.*

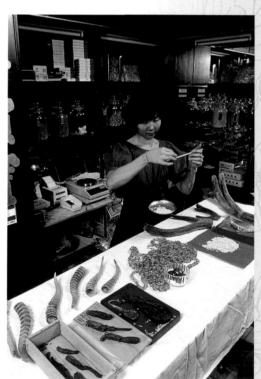

DRIED
ANGELICA ROOT

Angelica

ANGELICA ARCHANGELICA

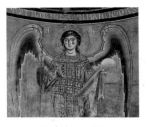

ABOVE *The Archangel Raphael
is said to have revealed the
healing properties of angelica.*

*This stately plant is linked to the Archangel Raphael,
who is said to have appeared in a dream to a medieval
monk in the 10th century and revealed that the herb was
a cure for plague. From then on it was called angelica and used
as a first line of defense against the disease.*

General description

Also called garden angelica, the whole of this tall plant,
which has small green flowers arranged in large globular
umbels, has a pleasant, distinctive smell. Thought to
originate in the Near East, angelica is widely cultivated
for use in cookery and liqueurs and is often found
growing in the wild. The seeds, root, and stems are used.
There are some 70 species of angelica in the world, all
with much the same use, but check in local herbals first.

Actions and character

Circulatory stimulant, antispasmodic, carminative, bitter
tonic, antiseptic, expectorant, diuretic, diaphoretic,
emmenagog. Generally warming and strengthening.

PROFESSIONAL USES

Angelica is used in the
same manner as in the
home and there are no
current additional
professional uses.

CHEMICAL CONSTITUENTS

Volatile oil, bitters,
furanocoumarins, resin,
tannins.

DOMESTIC USES

The leaves make a
pleasant, aromatic
addition to salads. The
young stems may be
peeled and used as a
vegetable, but only in
small amounts because of
their strong taste. Regular
use of angelica is said to
create a distaste for
alcohol. The powdered
seeds may be used as an
insecticide, especially for
head lice; they work best
in sunshine. Recent
research has found that
angelica resists the spread
of cancer in the body.

RIGHT *A majestic plant,
angelica has large bright
green glossy leaves.*

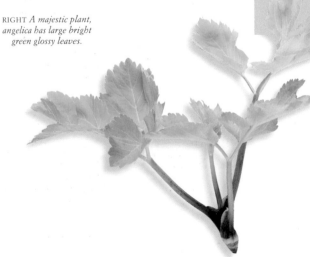

CAUTION

Do not use angelica
during pregnancy. The fresh
plant can occasionally cause
a rash when handled in
bright sunlight.

HOME USE

INTERNAL USES
• Indigestion, weak appetite, flatulence, liverishness, and colicky stomach pains.
• Period pains with delayed menstruation.
• Bronchitis and coughs with stubborn and infected phlegm.
• It is helpful in asthma.

• Sore throats, colds, flu, and fevers.
• Convalescence, general debility, chronic fatigue, feelings of great cold. A helpful general and digestive tonic for those with a cold constitution.

EXTERNAL USES
• The infused oil is used for massaging stiff joints and aching muscles.

DOSAGE

Use the seeds for digestive problems, chewed or taken as an infusion or tincture.

The stem and leaves have the mildest flavor and are considered more suitable for children, taken as an infusion or syrup.

Make a compress of the crushed root for headache and painful joints.

The root is the most restorative part, used by itself or with other roots for chronic weakness and cold conditions (see Elecampane, pp. 70–71). Decoction: use ½oz (15g) to 2½ cups (600ml) water, simmer 10 minutes in a covered vessel. Take 2 or 3 cups daily. Tincture: take 3 or 4 tsp (15 or 20ml) daily.

RELATED PLANTS

CHINESE ANGELICA

Chinese medicine uses several species of angelica, but the best known is Dang gui (Angelica sinensis), also called the "women's ginseng." It has the same uses as other angelicas but in addition is regarded as a specific tonic for debilitated women. It is very helpful for the following conditions: painful periods with a long cycle or slight blood flow, anemia, low blood pressure, and thick, white vaginal discharge. It is used as a restorative after giving birth and, with other herbs, for early menopause.

Various tablets are available and the herb is often included in food supplements with vitamins and minerals.

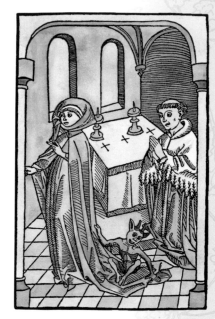

ABOVE *Angelica root juice was used as protection against witchcraft.*

RECIPE

Candied Angelica Stems

Candied angelica was originally made as a therapeutic cough lozenge. It is effective in warming and soothing the chest.

⚘ Cut the stems into 1-in (2.5-cm) lengths and simmer in sugar water until they are soft. ⚘ Strain. ⚘ Simmer again, in a sugar syrup, using 1 pound (450g) sugar in ¼ cups (300ml) water, for an hour. ⚘ Strain. ⚘ Let dry. ⚘ Sprinkle with confectioner's sugar and store in an airtight tin.

Dosage: chew a 2-in (5-cm) strip every few hours.

HISTORICAL NOTES

❀ Angelica was regarded by herbalists as an almost supernatural tonic and restorative. They used it to treat severe infectious fevers, including typhus, typhoid fever, and the plague, to cure the "bites of mad dogs," and to "resist poisons and witchcraft." Culpeper described it as "of admirable use."

❀ Native Americans used a compress of crushed angelica for pain and painful swellings. It was applied to the opposite side of the body and was said to draw the pain through the body before expelling it.

❀ Angelica roots were carried as a talisman for good luck in hunting.

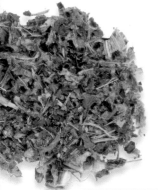

DRIED BURDOCK LEAVES

Burdock

ARCTIUM LAPPA

So named because of its seed heads, the burs, which are covered in hooks that catch onto passing animals or clothes; burdock is a familiar plant of waysides and wasteland. It has long been used as a general cleansing remedy.

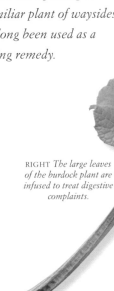

RIGHT *The large leaves of the burdock plant are infused to treat digestive complaints.*

General description

This stout, biennial plant has large leaves that are downy underneath. The flowers of the burdock are reddish-purple, occasionally white, and resemble thistle flowers. Found throughout the temperate regions of Eurasia and North America, the different species of burdock hybridize with each other and are difficult to tell apart. Fortunately they can all be used in medicine. The root, leaves, and seeds are used. Some herbalists prefer the whole seed heads, picked while still green.

Actions and character

Alterative, blood cleanser, bitter tonic, antibiotic, lymphatic cleanser, diuretic, diaphoretic. Mild laxative and nutritive (root).

PROFESSIONAL USES

Cancer, chronic hepatitis, protective in immune deficiencies including H.I.V. infection.

RECIPE

Pickled Burdock Stalks

Pickled burdock is a traditional Japanese food used to accompany rice dishes. Adding the spices brings out the sweetness and makes it more versatile as well as strengthening its valued aphrodisiac qualities.

Quantity of young leaf stalks (these are best picked in early summer)

☙ Peel and chop into even lengths, and blanch in boiling water.

☙ To each cup of burdock stalks use:

- *1 cup cider vinegar*
- *2 tbsp (30ml) sugar*
- *½ tsp (2ml) powdered cinnamon*
- *A good pinch of powdered cloves*

☙ Loosely fill a pickle jar with the burdock. Put the other ingredients into a pan and bring to a boil, stir, and pour over the burdock. Fill into jars and seal.

CAUTION

Burdock is generally safe to use, but it is best to avoid large doses in pregnancy. Burdock may cause a temporary exacerbation of symptoms. If this proves inconvenient, lower the dose and consider seeking professional advice for proper support.

DOMESTIC USES

The large leaves make excellent emergency hats for those unexpectedly caught out by rain on long country hikes.

CHEMICAL CONSTITUENTS

Bitters, flavonoids, tannins, trace of volatile oil. Fatty oils (seeds). Inulin and mucilage (roots).

HOME USE

DOSAGE

Burdock is best used in fairly small doses over a long period.

The root or seeds are decocted; the leaf is infused. Take 2 cups of tea a day for six months. Decoction: 1oz (25g) daily. Tincture: 2 or 3 tsp (10 or 15ml) daily.

Burdock is traditionally combined with other herbs; with dandelion root for arthritis and skin diseases; with yellow dock root for psoriasis and other stubborn skin diseases; with echinacea for boils and infected skin conditions.

The seeds are used in Chinese medicine for sore throats and viral infections with an unproductive cough.

Regular drinking of a decoction of the seeds is said to restore skin tone and smoothness. They are also of benefit in cases of sciatica.

INTERNAL USES

• The leaves and the green seed heads are the most bitter parts and most suitable for digestive problems and acute skin problems.
• Arthritis, rheumatism, and gout.
• Skin diseases: acne, spots, boils, eczema, and psoriasis. As a skin wash for infected spots.
• Chronic constipation.
 • Weak digestion and poor appetite.
• Mouth ulcers, as a tea and mouthwash.
• Helps reduce cholesterol levels.
• For water retention, when used in combination with dandelion.

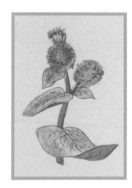

BURDOCK

BELOW Use burdock regularly for its cleansing, antiseptic, and strengthening properties.

HISTORICAL NOTES

❀ This cleansing remedy of traditional medicine was used to expel any sort of poison from the system. The 17th-century herbalist Nicholas Culpeper recommends the leaves as a compress for "shrunken sinews," the seed drunk in wine for sciatica, and the candied root for "consumption."

❀ Recent research reports an anti-tumor action, and burdock is included in the folk remedy "Essiac."

❀ In his play *As You Like It*, Shakespeare refers to the "holiday foolery" of throwing the burs so they catch on people's clothing.

❀ In the north of England dandelion and burdock was a traditional cordial. It had the same tonic, cleansing, and strengthening qualities of the original sarsaparilla or cola. It is still available as a soft drink, but it bears little resemblance to the original cordial and contains none of the beneficial qualities.

❀ The root is eaten in the East, as a vegetable and to strengthen failing sexual powers in older people. In Europe the peeled, young stalks were cooked and eaten like asparagus for the same reasons.

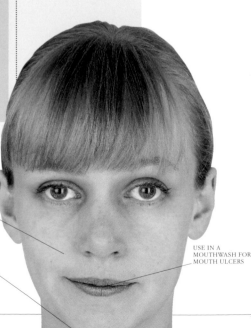

RESTORES SKIN TONE AND SMOOTHNESS

RELIEVES SORE THROATS

USE IN A MOUTHWASH FOR MOUTH ULCERS

45

Mugwort

ARTEMESIA VULGARIS

DRIED
MUGWORT
FLOWERS

*In the Middle Ages mugwort was considered a magical protective herb,
effective against witches and the Devil. It grows alongside paths and
trails, and was traditionally thought to accompany travelers providing
the help to strengthen and protect those on their "life-path."*

General description

Mugwort is a medium to tall, rather hairy, and aromatic
plant with deeply cut leaves. The flowers are very small,
reddish-brown, and often not noticed. It is common on
wasteland and waysides throughout Eurasia and
America. In North America other species of artemesia
are also called mugwort. They have much the same uses.
The whole herb is used, especially the tops, picked just
as they come into flower.

Actions and character

Gently stimulating nervine, emmenagog,
menstrual regulator, diaphoretic, cholagog,
bitter tonic.

BELOW *Chew a little
mugwort when hiking
to fight fatigue.*

PROFESSIONAL USES

Epilepsy, Parkinson's
disease, infertility.

DOMESTIC USES

Mugwort and related
species are used to make
moxa sticks for Chinese
medicine. They may also
be bound up into smudge
sticks to use for ritual
cleansing of people
and places.
Placed under the pillow,
mugwort will bring focus
to dreams and help
protect against
nightmares.
Mugwort promotes the
appetite and may be
added to stews and
stuffing for meat dishes.
Use as an insect repellent.
Moths and other insects
are said to dislike the
mugwort plant.
The flower remedy is used
to promote awareness and
to "rebalance" psychic
awareness.

LEFT *The aromatic
mugwort was one of
the nine sacred herbs
of the Anglo-Saxons.*

HOME USE

INTERNAL USES
• Delayed and painful menstruation. Irregular menstruation with light flow of blood.
• Early stages of colds and fevers.
• Indigestion with poor appetite and cramps.
• As an aperitif.
• Liverishness with nausea and heavy headaches.
• Depression with liver or digestive disorders.
• Nervousness in run-down or debilitated people.
• Useful remedy for arthritis and gout.
• Intestinal worms.

EXTERNAL USES
• The vinegar on a compress is useful for bruises or swollen and inflamed joints.

DOSAGE

By infusion: one or two cups daily. Take half a cup every 4 hours for fevers.

Tincture: ½–1 tsp (2–5ml) three times daily.

Three or four of the fresh leaves, chewed slowly, for fatigue. When tired on a country hike, look for some mugwort by the path. Pick a few leaves or flowering tops, and chew them thoroughly. Your tiredness will dissipate and the path seem easier as the bitter aromatics clear the mind and eyes.

RECIPE

Smudge Sticks

These can be made from any species of artemesia.

☙ Pick the tops of the herbs, just before the flowers open. ☙ Pick pieces of the same length, about 6in (15cm) long. ☙ Let dry for a day or two. ☙ Gather into a bundle about 1in (2.5cm) across and bind together with cotton thread. ☙ Do not use synthetic fiber. ☙ To use, set fire to the end, blow out the flame, and let smolder.

BELOW *Weary travelers placed mugwort in their shoes as a remedy against tired, aching feet.*

HISTORICAL NOTES

❧ Mugwort has long been used to revive weary travelers and to protect them against evil spirits and attack by wild beasts. Roman soldiers placed it in their shoes to help aching feet. William Coles in *The Art of Simpling* (1656) says, "If a footman put it into his shoes in the morning, he may goe 40 miles before noon and not be weary."

❧ Mugwort was called sailor's or poor man's tobacco and used by itself or with other herbs in smoking mixtures. It was also used to flavor beer at one time.

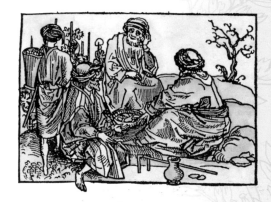

RELATED PLANTS

There are some 200 species of artemesia in the world, all with similar uses but of varying strengths. It is difficult to tell them apart and expert local knowledge may be required. Mugwort is the mildest and safest for home use. Wormwood (Artemesia absinthium) is generally regarded as the strongest. Small amounts of wormwood herb are used to flavor vermouth and other aperitif drinks. Sweet wormwood (Artemesia annua) is used in China and Africa to treat malaria. In North America artemesias are sometimes called "sage" or "sagebrush" which can be a source of confusion. They are not related to garden sage (Salvia officinalis).

CAUTION

Do not take in pregnancy or when breast-feeding. Do not take for long periods of time without professional advice.

CHEMICAL CONSTITUENTS

Essential oil, bitter sesquiterpenes, flavonoids, tannins, resin.

Cabbage

BRASSICA OLERACEA (BRASSICA SYLVESTRIS)

The cabbage is not only a useful vegetable but an invaluable plant
in herbal medicine. Many remedies can be prepared simply from
any of the varieties available. Internally, its main use is to cleanse
the system; externally, the leaves make a good poultice to help
reduce hot swellings.

General description

Wild cabbage is regarded as a
native of southern England and
the coasts of the Mediterranean and
Adriatic. When found elsewhere it is
considered as an escapee. It is a dark
green, stringy version of its cultivated
brethren. Selective cultivation has highlighted
various features of the plant, rewarding us with
white, red, and green cabbage, Savoy, kale, Brussels
sprouts, cauliflower, kohlrabi, broccoli, and calabrese –
all have the same basic properties.

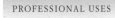

ABOVE *There are now many*
different varieties of cultivated
cabbage plants. They can all be
used in herbal remedies.

Actions and character

Cooling, soothing, slightly demulcent. Nutritive.
Detoxifying, alkalizes the body, mildly laxative.

R E C I P E

Sauerkraut

German for sour cabbage,
sauerkraut retains the
nutritional properties of
cabbage. It was traditionally
eaten in the winter, when
fresh fruit and vegetables
were not available.
Fermenting cabbage is an
exacting process, but it
makes an excellent relish.

⚘ Use 2 tsp (10ml) salt for
every 5 cups (1lb/500g)
thinly sliced cabbage. Mix
together and pack firmly
into a container, cover

with a cloth, and hold down
with a weight. ⚘ When
fermentation starts, remove
the scum daily. ⚘ Keep the
cloth clean and the
temperature below 60°F
(16°C). Fermentation takes
about a month. ⚘ When
finished, bring the cabbage
to a boil for a moment, pack
into jars, cover with a weak
brine, and seal.

Dosage (as a supplement):
1 tbsp (15ml) daily in soups,
broth, casseroles, or with
cold meats.

PROFESSIONAL USES

The juice as a soothing
demulcent for stomach
and bowel cancer.

DOMESTIC USES

Poultices: use whole
leaves and remove the
middle rib if it is very
thick. Blanch or
soften leaves and wrap
them around the body.
Cover with plastic
wrap or a light crêpe
bandage to keep in place.
Leave overnight. To
reduce swelling, repeat
every 4 hours or until
the swelling subsides.

HOME USE

INTERNAL USES
• Cooling in fevers.
• Strong cabbage water and honey helps soothe a child's cough.
• For ulcers, gastritis, and heartburn.
• After overindulgence one or two days of light diet and cabbage water is less stressful than a fast.
• Helps alkalize the body when it is too acidic, gouty, or arthritic; good for cystitis.
• Cuts fats and aids digestion.

EXTERNAL USES
• Cabbage water on hot itchy or irritable skin conditions. Cabbage juice for mild burns, sunburn, and cold sores.
• For swollen joints, any hot swelling, drawing abscesses, and reducing pain in sprains. Sore breasts and sore throats.

DOSAGE

Cabbage water as a decoction. Use 1 cup thinly sliced cabbage to 4 cups water. Simmer for 10 minutes and strain. Drink freely, or take ¼–½ cup twice a day. For a warming element a pinch of spice may be added. Coriander, cumin, nutmeg, mace, and allspice are all traditional accompaniments.

As a cleanser and rebalancer, mix 1 cup chopped sweet apples, 1 cup chopped cabbage, 1 tsp (5ml) caraway seed, 3 cups water. Simmer over a very low heat for 10 minutes. Strain the liquid, add more water to make back up to 3 cups liquid. Drink freely throughout the day.

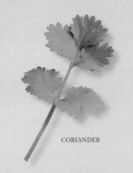

CORIANDER

HISTORICAL NOTES

Cabbage has long been used as medicine and food. Culpeper (1653) sings its medicinal praises: "Boiled in broth and eaten, opens the body [mild laxative] ... eaten with meat it keeps one from surfeiting, and from getting drunk [coats stomach, cuts fats, adds bulky dietary fiber] ... drink and bathe the joints for pain, aches, and gouty swellings. Heals all small scabs, pulses, and wheels that break out in the skin [cooling, cleanser, and detoxifier internally and externally] ... for melancholy and windy humors."

The workers who built the Great Wall of China were fed a type of fermented Chinese cabbage to keep them strong and healthy.

CHEMICAL CONSTITUENTS

High in minerals including calcium, potassium, sulphur, silica, magnesium, and iron. (Weight for weight, cabbage contains more calcium than milk.) Vitamins A, B, C, and E. Mucilage and mustard oils.

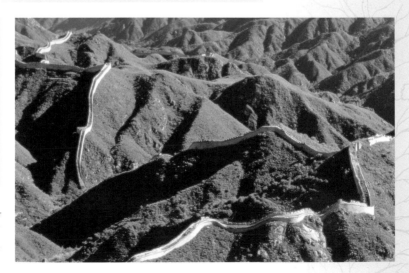

RIGHT *The Great Wall of China, one of the world's greatest feats of engineering, was built by workers fed on a diet of fermented cabbage.*

Marigold

CALENDULA OFFICINALIS

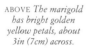

DRIED
MARIGOLD
FLOWERS

*The old name for this annual garden
plant was "golds," because of its large, bright
yellow or orange flowers. This plant has earned its place
in traditional gardens by being both an invaluable home
remedy, internally and externally, and an ingredient in
cooking. The plant is also called pot marigold, from its use in
cooking.*

ABOVE *The marigold
has bright golden
yellow petals, about
3in (7cm) across.*

General description

This common garden plant was originally from southern
Europe but is easily grown in temperate and warm, dry
climates. It likes a sunny position and will happily grow
in window boxes and pots. The flowers are used in
herbal medicine – choose bright orange flowers for the
best medicine. Marigold preparations are easily available
to buy, and are often called Calendula.

Actions and character

Immune tonic, lymphatic deobstructant, antiseptic,
styptic, anti-inflammatory, antifungal. Healing and
uplifting properties.

PROFESSIONAL USES

Douche and pessaries for
precancerous conditions
of the vagina and cervix.
Internal use as an adjunct
in treating breast cancer,
inflamed tumors in
general, endometriosis,
and ovarian cysts.

DOMESTIC USES

Marigold petals are
traditionally added to
broth and stews to make
them more nourishing.
A few flowers add depth
of flavor to vegetarian
soups and casseroles. You
can sprinkle the petals
into rice before cooking,
instead of saffron, or add
them to salads. A yellow
dye may be extracted
from the flowers. The
essential oil is a good
anti-inflammatory, but
difficult to obtain and
expensive. For most cases
the infused oil proves a
good alternative.

CAUTION

Do not confuse with Tagetes species.
These are the French, African, and Aztec
marigolds, which have different properties
and should not be used internally. They can,
however, be used in ointments for corns and
are often planted around vegetables
to keep pests away.

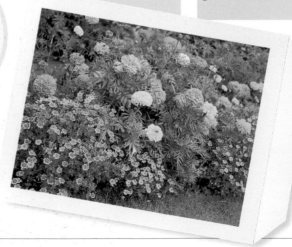

RIGHT *Popular for their bright
yellow blooms and long
flowering season, French,
African and Aztec marigolds
should never be used internally.*

HOME USE

EXTERNAL USE
• The single most useful remedy for skin diseases, especially inflamed and infected wounds, cuts, broken chilblains, and infected skin rashes.
• Use the tincture to dry and heal spots, sores, cuts, bruises, ringworm, and other fungal infections.
• Use the cream for rashes, varicose veins, raw and chapped skin, itchy anus, thrush, and as a lip balm. Use the infused oil on dry, scaly rashes such as cradle cap.

• A marigold compress will help bring down an inflammation. Make a compress from marigold tea or tincture for inflamed cuts, boils, sore nipples, and also sore eyes.
• Use with witch hazel for painful varicose veins.

DOSAGE
May be taken freely.

For children's fevers, three or four marigold flowerheads infused in a cup of boiling water, ½ cup every 2 hours.

For compresses, infuse a handful of marigold flowers in a pint of hot water for 15 minutes.

INTERNAL USE
• Use a strong tea or diluted tincture as a mouthwash or gargle for painful gum disease and sore throats.
• Take tea or tincture for swollen lymph nodes (swollen glands), mumps, children's fevers, chronic tonsillitis, gastritis, gallbladder problems, painful periods, cellulite, and for promoting healing after any operations.
• Use with comfrey for adhesions and stomach ulcers and with sage to prevent flu.

HISTORICAL NOTES
Aemilius Macer, writing in the 13th century, says that simply gazing on the flowers draws "wicked humors out of the head" and "makes the sight bright and clean."

The sight and smell of marigolds is very cheering and uplifting, and they have long been recommended to "comfort the heart" and to "protect it in fevers."

RECIPE
Marigold Pudding

• 1 handful of marigold petals
• 1 cup (4oz/125g) flour
• 2 cups (4oz/125g) soft bread crumbs
• 1 tsp (5ml) baking powder
• ¼ tsp (2ml) salt
• ½ cup (4oz/125g) chopped suet
• ¼ cup (2oz/60g) sugar
• Sufficient milk to mix (about ⅔ cup [2oz/150ml])

Mix the dry ingredients together in a basin. Stir in the milk a little at a time, until a soft dropping consistency is obtained. Turn into a greased basin and steam for at least 2 hours. Serve with a sweet sauce.

CHEMICAL CONSTITUENTS
Resin, small amount of essential oil, flavonoids, mucilage, saponins.

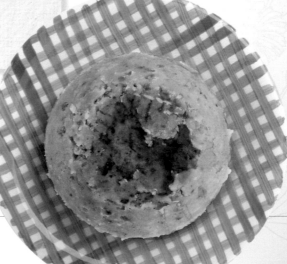

RIGHT *Use marigold petals to make a nutritious and tasty steamed pudding.*

Cayenne pepper

CAPSICUM MINIMUM AND OTHER SPECIES

Best known as the familiar, red, hot-tasting kitchen spice
that is also called capsicum, red pepper, or chili pepper,
cayenne is used medicinally mainly as a general stimulant
and to build up resistance at the beginning of a cold.

LEFT *Cayenne powder is a popular spice in the kitchen as well as in herbal medicine.*

CHEMICAL CONSTITUENTS

Volatile oil, flavonoids, alkaloids including capsaicin, vitamin C.

PROFESSIONAL USES

Cayenne is used in the same manner as in the home and there are no current additional professional uses.

General description

The ripe fruit of this woody, tropical plant is the part used in herbal medicine. Originally from Central America but now grown all over the world, cayenne pepper is essential to the culinary traditions of many countries. Many varieties are available and the "hotness" is variable. Some varieties of cayenne can be grown in temperate climates if sown under glass early in the year.

DOMESTIC USES

Add pepper to foods that are hard to digest or that provoke wind.

Actions and character

Diaphoretic, antispasmodic, carminative, a strong circulatory stimulant, digestive tonic, antiseptic, anodyne.

LEFT *Fresh red chilies, the source of the hot, pungent cayenne pepper.*

RECIPE
Hot Oil

- 2 tsp (10ml) cayenne pepper
- 4 tsp (20ml) of powdered mustard seed
- 2 tsp (10ml) powdered ginger root
- 2 cups unblended vegetable, sunflower, or grape seed oil.

Hot oil is an infused oil, so called because it is hot to the taste. It is a warming antispasmodic rub, improving circulation and relaxing muscle tension and spasm. Use for massaging into knotted muscles and aching joints. Do not use over large areas of the body.

CAUTION

Do not use cayenne with an acid stomach. Avoid large doses in pregnancy. It should be used with caution by hot people, in high fevers, in high blood pressure, and in inflammatory gut conditions. It is more suitable for adults, including the elderly, than children. Be sure to wash your hands after handling cayenne.

HOME USE

- Cayenne is a versatile and valuable home remedy, but it must be used in small amounts.

INTERNAL USES
- Beneficial if added to any herbal prescription for circulatory complaints, for people with poor circulation, or for people frightened of the cold.
- Low stomach acidity, indigestion with flatulence and bloating.
- Loss of appetite after fevers or in elderly people.
- A weak gargle for sore throats and loss of voice.

EXTERNAL USES
- Locally in creams, liniments, and plasters for poor circulation, cold feet, neuralgia and post-shingles neuralgia, back pains, lumbago, and sciatica. Unbroken chilblains (use marigold on broken chilblains).

DOSAGE

Cayenne is usually added to other remedies.

A very small pinch of cayenne powder can be added to herbal teas, such as yarrow or elderflower, for colds and fevers.

A homemade tincture is simply made, by soaking the fresh or dried peppers in vodka for a few days. Take 3–4 drops in herbal tea or warm water three or four times daily. Those people who wish to avoid alcohol can substitute vinegar.

For prostration, repeat the dose every few hours until feeling better.

For lumbago and chronic back pain, add cayenne tincture to a liniment – ¼ tsp (1ml) cayenne tincture to ¼ tsp (3ml) liniment. Apply sparingly and cover with plastic. Leave on for a half hour. Repeat daily.

An effective country treatment for cold feet is to sprinkle red pepper inside the socks.

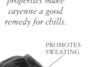
BELOW *Its warming properties make cayenne a good remedy for chills.*

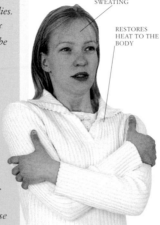

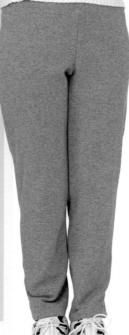

PROMOTES SWEATING

RESTORES HEAT TO THE BODY

Cayenne was popularized by the U.S. herbalist Samuel Thompson (1769–1843) as a sure and simple cure for the dangerous fevers prevalent in those days. He recommended large doses to sweat the fever out. This is a strategy more suitable for strong constitutions and severe, acute fevers. These days weaker constitutions and chronic diseases are more the rule but cayenne still has its place, in smaller doses, to "restore the vital heat of the body."

In recent years creams made from cayenne and its alkaloid, capsaicin, have been used in hospitals as a painkiller.

SIMILAR PLANTS

Ginger (Zingiber officinale) is a suitable warming remedy for people who find cayenne too hot. It is more diffusive than cayenne and easier on the digestion, more suitable for the onset of chills, for period pains, and for gut spasms. Ginger is specific for nausea, travel sickness, and the nausea of pregnancy. Traditionally it was used to revive a lowered sex drive, and add a warm, stimulant spice to life. Make a tincture with fresh root and vodka; take 10–30 drops in hot water or herbal teas, or add to other tinctures.

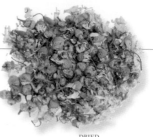

Camomile

CHAMOMILLA RECUTITA

According to the ancient Anglo-Saxon text, the Lacnunga, *camomile was one of the nine sacred herbs given to the world by the god Woden. Also known as German camomile or* Matricaria chamomilla, *camomile is widely cultivated and is used to make one of the most popular herbal teas in the world.*

General description

Growing up to 2ft (60cm), the German camomile has small daisy-like white flowers. The bright green feathery leaves have an apple-like scent. This annual plant is found wild in most temperate regions, growing in fields and along roadsides. The flowers are used medicinally as a tonic and sedative.

Actions and character

Relaxant, sedative, antispasmodic, anti-inflammatory, anti-allergic. Soothing and calming.

ABOVE *German camomile has delicate apple-scented white flowers.*

DOMESTIC USES

Camomile is a gentle bleach, often contained in shampoos for lightening hair, and the tea can be used as a hair rinse. The best-quality essential oil is blue, from the azulenes. It is expensive but worth the extra cost.

Homeopathic preparations, called chamomilla, have the same properties and may be easier to give to children. Use the flower remedy to relieve emotional tension and as an aid to meditation.

PROFESSIONAL USES

Inhalants for asthma.

BELOW *Camomile is used to lighten hair, and is found in many hair-care preparations.*

RELATED PLANTS

*Roman or English camomile (*Anthemis noblis*) is a perennial with the same properties as wild camomile. It tastes a little bitter and is therefore not such a pleasant tea to drink, but the whole plant is very aromatic. A non-flowering variety of this species, lawn camomile, is, as its name suggests, planted as a lawn for the wonderful fragrance that it releases when walked on. In Henry IV Part 1, Shakespeare refers to it: "The more it is trodden on, the more it grows." At one time raised beds of lawn camomile were used as seats, not only for their pleasant scent but also to relieve the pain of piles. Do not take this camomile during pregnancy.*

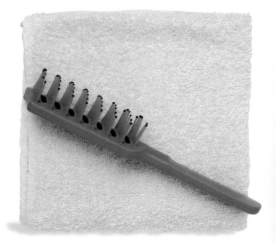

HOME USE

EXTERNAL USE
• Infused oil, creams, and compresses for irritable and itchy skin conditions including eczema. A few drops of the volatile oil may be added to creams for the same uses.
• The vinegar for itchy conditions of the genitals or on sensitive skin.
• Inhalants for hay fever.
• Use as a compress for tired and sore eyes and allergic reactions.
• Poultices and warm compresses for any sort of spasmodic pain.

INTERNAL USE
• The tea is safe for infants and useful for insomnia, nightmares, over-excitability, and teething problems.

DOSAGE

An excellent drinking tea for stress management, to be taken frequently. Make a double-strength tea for medicinal use and use a covered vessel in order to prevent all the goodness escaping in the steam.

Two cups of camomile tea in the bath water will soothe restless infants.

• Calms the digestive system. Nervous indigestion, wind, colic pains, gastritis, and inflammation of the digestive tract.
• Mildly sedative. Good for stress headaches, psychosomatic conditions, period pains, and other spasmodic pains.
• Useful in the early stages of fever.
• The tincture is best for nervous indigestion.
• Camomile and rosemary is a good combination tea to take for headaches.

HISTORICAL NOTES

✂ Camomile was used by the Ancient Egyptians and large amounts are still grown in Egypt for home use and export.

✂ Camomile pollen was found in the mummified stomach of Rameses II.

✂ The Anglo-Saxons called it maythen and numbered it among their most sacred herbs.

✂ The name camomile itself comes from the ancient Greek word meaning "ground apple," on account of its apple-like scent, although this probably refers to the Roman camomile.

✂ Parkinson's *Herbal* of 1656 recommends camomile baths, to "comfort and strengthen the sound and to ease pains in the diseased."

RECIPE

Relaxing Tea

🌿 Mix together equal parts of camomile flowers, linden flowers, lemon balm (melissa) or lemon verbena 🌿 Make a tea in the usual way (see p. 24).

This is a useful and pleasant drinking tea, especially for people who find camomile lacking in flavor. Take freely to help cope with stress.

RIGHT Camomile is one of the safest herbs and may be used to soothe restless children.

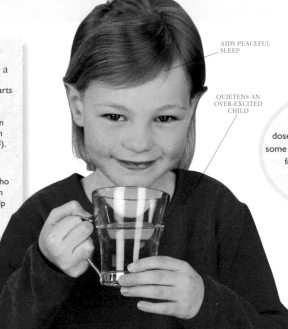

AIDS PEACEFUL SLEEP

QUIETENS AN OVER-EXCITED CHILD

CAUTION

Although camomile is safe, large doses and strong teas can cause nausea in some people. Avoid large doses in pregnancy for this reason. Some people have a contact allergy to fresh camomile.

CHEMICAL CONSTITUENTS

Volatile oil, bitter principles including azulene, flavonoids, malic acid.

Cinnamon

CINNAMOMUM ZEYLANICUM AND CINNAMOMUM CASSIA

Dried cinnamon bark (C. zeylanicum), rolled into small cylindrical bundles called quills, is a popular cooking spice around the world. The cinnamon twigs of C. cassia are often used in medicine. They are less pungent than the bark and more gently warming.

CINNAMON POWDER

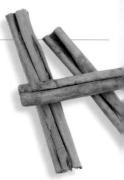

ABOVE *The inner bark of the cinnamon tree is rolled into sticks.*

General description

The cinnamon is a large tree originating in southeast Asia but now widely grown in tropical countries. The bark is collected from the mature shoots of the trees.

Actions and character

Warming, antispasmodic, carminative, astringent, antiseptic.

PROFESSIONAL USES

Cinnamon is used professionally in the same manner as in the home and there are no additional uses.

DOMESTIC USES

The aromatic, slightly sweet taste of cinnamon bark makes it a popular spice to add to cakes and cookies and, of course, apple pie.
Essential oils of both species are available and widely used in aromatherapy for aches and pains, depression, and loss of interest in life. They can be irritating to sensitive skins and must be well diluted. A few drops can be added to liniments for rheumatism and muscle pains with much benefit.

RECIPE

Cinnamon Toast

This is a pleasant way of taking cinnamon and a useful addition to the diet in cold weather.

- 2 tsps (10ml) powdered cinnamon
- Small pinch ground nutmeg (optional)
- 4 tbsp (60g) granulated brown sugar
- 3 tbsp (45g) butter

☞ Mash the spices, sugar, and butter together and spread onto thinly sliced whole-wheat bread. ☞ Put under a very hot broiler until the sugar caramelizes.

Eat two or three slices for breakfast every morning.

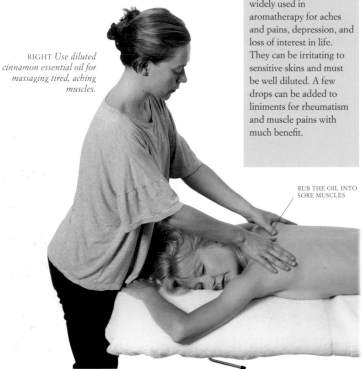

RIGHT *Use diluted cinnamon essential oil for massaging tired, aching muscles.*

RUB THE OIL INTO SORE MUSCLES

HOME USE

INTERNAL USES
• Chills, colds, and fevers.
• Coughs.
• As a tea or massage oil for poor circulation.
• Good for exhaustion and feelings of cold following severe illness or prolonged stress.
• Indigestion and weak digestion with wind and griping pains.
• Diarrhea.
• Irritable bowel.

EXTERNAL USES
• Head and body lice.
• Mouthwash for gum disease and gargle for tonsillitis. Included in toothpastes.

DOSAGE

For coughs, colds, and fevers add a good pinch of powdered cinnamon to any suitable herbal tea, or make a tincture in vodka and add 20 drops to the herb tea.

For colds with a running nose, chew a short piece of the bark.

Combines well with ginger for chills, nausea, and indigestion.

For head lice, add 20 drops of the essential oil to the final rinsing water after washing your hair. May also be used as a preventive.

CAUTION

Do not use in pregnancy as a medicinal dosage can be stimulative. Culinary use is safe.

HISTORICAL NOTES

✿ Cinnamon was known to the ancient Egyptians who added it to their best perfumes and used it in the spice mixtures for wrapping mummies.

✿ It is still used in Arab countries as a warming drink in cold weather.

✿ In Indian medicine it was traditionally used to strengthen the system, promote digestion, and aid the absorption of other remedies.

✿ Traditional Chinese medicine uses the twigs for cold hands and feet and cinnamon bark for warming the trunk.

✿ British "digestive biscuits," made from soothing oats, were once also made with warming and carminative herbs such as cinnamon, ginger, and allspice, and were eaten specifically to aid digestion. Today they have lost this function.

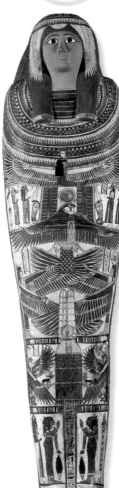

LEFT *The Ancient Egyptians used cinnamon in their funerary practices.*

RECIPE
Parfait Amour

This is a traditional French aphrodisiac liqueur.

• 6-in (15-cm) piece of cinnamon quill
• 1 tbsp (15ml) fresh or dried thyme
• ¼ vanilla bean
• 1 tsp (5ml) coriander seeds
• ½ tsp (2ml) powdered mace
• Peel from 1 small lemon
• 2½ cups (600ml) good-quality brandy
• ⅓ cup (8oz/250g) honey
• 1¼ cups (300ml) water

✿ Crush the dry ingredients together using a mortar and pestle or a coffee grinder.
✿ Add to the brandy and leave in a cool place for two weeks, shaking from time to time.
✿ Strain.
✿ Warm the water and dissolve the honey in it.
✿ Add to the spiced brandy.
✿ Bottle and label.
✿ Dosage: 3 tbsp (45ml) before bed.

CHEMICAL CONSTITUENTS

Essential oil, tannins.

Hawthorn

CRATAEGUS OXYACANTHOIDES, CRATAEGUS MONOGYNA

*Also called whitethorn, or May, from its flowering time, this common hedgerow
tree has been shown by research to have a beneficial effect on the heart –
it relaxes and dilates the coronary arteries, thus improving blood flow to the heart.*

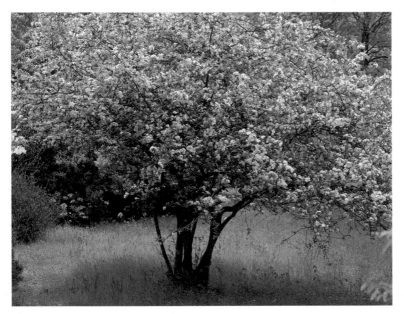

ABOVE *The hawthorn tree can
grow up to 30ft (9m) high. In
the late spring highly scented
white flowers appear on its
thorny branches. Red berries
follow in the fall.*

PROFESSIONAL USES

Coronary artery disease,
angina, heart failure,
hypertension,
arteriosclerosis; may be
used as a restorative after
heart attacks.

DOMESTIC USES

Properly layered
hawthorn hedges, made
by cutting halfway
through the young trees
and bending them over,
provide an excellent
habitat for wildlife and a
higher yield of flowers and
fruit than those hedges
made by using hedge
cutters.

The berries can be added
to crab apple jelly and
used to make wine.

General description

Hawthorn is a small, thorny tree bearing masses of white
blossom in late spring and red berries in the fall. Found
throughout northern, temperate regions, it is commonly
used as a hedging plant. A variety with double, red
flowers is often grown as an ornamental tree in parks
and gardens. The flowering tops (flowers and leaves) or
the berries are used.

The name whitethorn is in contrast to the blackthorn
or sloe, which flowers on bare branches. Some Asian
species of hawthorn are grown for their edible fruit.

DRIED
HAWTHORN TOPS

CHEMICAL CONSTITUENTS

Flavonoids including rutin,
tannins, saponins,
cyanogenic glycosides.

Actions and character

Heart restorative, relaxes and dilates the coronary
and peripheral arteries.

HOME USE

INTERNAL USES
• Indigestion with flatulence, colic, and feelings of fullness.
• Weak heart and poor circulation in the elderly, mildly increased blood pressure (without medication).
• Good for poor circulation in general.
• Raynaud's phenomenon.
• Fast heartbeat and palpitations. Fear of heart disease.

DOSAGE

An infusion of the flowering tops or a decoction of the berries, one cup twice daily. Needs to be taken for several months for maximum benefit. For mildly raised blood pressure and raised cholesterol levels, follow sensible dietary advice as well.

With valerian for palpitations from anxiety. For panic attacks mix the two tinctures in equal parts and carry a dropper bottle with you. Dose: 30 drops.

For emotional strain affecting the heart, and for a "broken heart," combine with skullcap.

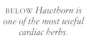

RIGHT *If you suffer from palpitations or anxiety, try using a tincture of valerian and hawthorn.*

BELOW *Hawthorn is one of the most useful cardiac herbs.*

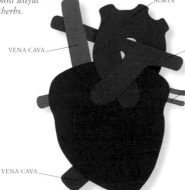

AORTA
VENA CAVA
PULMONARY ARTERY
PULMONARY VEINS
VENA CAVA

RECIPE
Hawthorn Berry Catsup

• 1½lb (750g) ripe berries
• 2 cups (450ml) cider vinegar
• ½ cup (4oz/125g) sugar
• 1 tsp (5ml) salt
• 2 tsp (10ml) allspice (pimento berries)

Cook the berries in the vinegar for about 20 minutes until soft. Press the pulp through a sieve with the back of a spoon, to extract the stones. Return to the pan, add the other ingredients and heat gently for 10 minutes longer. Store in sealed, sterilized bottles.

CAUTION

Hawthorn is safe to use, but if you are taking drugs for high blood pressure or heart problems, consult a professional herbalist first. People suffering from heart disease should be under the care of a professional.

HISTORICAL NOTES

Hawthorn was traditionally used for digestive pain and diarrhea – Chinese hawthorn berries (*Crataegus pinnatifida*) are still mostly used for this particular purpose.

Culpeper recommended the seeds in the berries, powdered and drunk in wine, as "good against the stone and dropsy."

In the last 100 years or so hawthorn has been mostly used for its beneficial effect on the heart, which has been proved by scientific research in Germany.

Traditionally hawthorn flowers were not brought into the house as they presaged death but they were taken to weddings as a symbol of good luck.

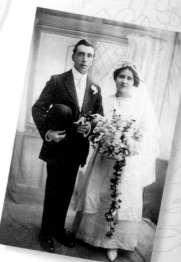

RIGHT *Hawthorn flowers were given to newly married couples for good luck.*

DRIED ECHINACEA ROOT

Echinacea

ECHINACEA ANGUSTIFOLIA, ECHINACEA PURPUREA

Native to North America, echinacea, commonly known as the coneflower, has long been used to treat infections. Recent research has validated traditional claims about its effectiveness, and the remedy has achieved widespread publicity as a herbal antibiotic. Echinacea has a tingling taste – the more tingle, the better the remedy.

General description

Echinacea has large, purple, late-flowering daisies with the same high, central cone as its close relatives, the rudbeckias. It grows best on chalk or limestone. The root, or sometimes the whole plant, is used. The green, unripe seeds also make good medicine. Echinacea has a strong, numbing taste.

Actions and character

Stimulates immune system response, antibiotic, lymphatic deobstructant, anti-inflammatory.

PROFESSIONAL USES

Septicemia, immune deficiencies, and to replace conventional antibiotics in a large number of conditions.

DOMESTIC USES

A handsome addition to most gardens, echinacea can be grown from seed or propagated from root cuttings. Different colored forms are available. Some herbalists think that *Echinacea purpurea* is more gentle than *angustifolia*.

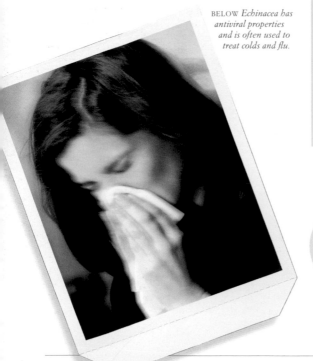

BELOW *Echinacea has antiviral properties and is often used to treat colds and flu.*

LEFT *The purple daisy-like flowers of the echinacea plant appear in late summer.*

CAUTION

Echinacea is safe to use, but be sure to take a large enough dose for acute conditions and to use together with more restorative herbs in chronic conditions. Use in immune-deficiency conditions only with professional guidance.

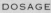

ECHINACEA TABLETS

HOME USE

INTERNAL USES
• Infections in general; sore throats, mouth ulcers, gum disease, tooth abscess, blocked salivary glands, and fevers following vaccinations.
• Strengthens resistance to infection, prophylactic for those suffering from recurrent minor infections. Suitable for children continually suffering from tonsillitis, ear infections, colds, and other minor infections.
• Skin diseases; boils, acne, abscesses, and eczema with hot, red skin.
• Duodenal and stomach ulcers.
• Herpes.
• Helpful in allergies.
• Depression with exhaustion.
• May be used in conjunction with antibiotics.

EXTERNAL USES
• As a douche for vaginal infections and a wash for infected wounds.

RIGHT *Children suffering from minor infections can safely take echinacea.*

DOSAGE

A common mistake with echinacea is not to take a sufficient quantity.

For acute infections such as tonsillitis, tooth abscesses, and genital herpes, take a cup of the decoction or 2 tsp (10ml) of tincture every 4 to 6 hours for up to 10 days.

For chronic conditions and long-term use, combine with less stimulating cleansing or restorative herbs – for example, with marigold and burdock for skin conditions, with sage for persistent infections, sore throats, and post-viral exhaustion.

Echinacea is also excellent for local application: use the decoction as a gargle for infected sore throats, as a mouthwash for gum infections, and to numb the pain of toothache.

Tablets and capsules are widely available; follow the instructions on the package. Garlic and echinacea is an effective combination for treating winter infections. Coated tablets containing 50mg echinacea extract are effective for, and well tolerated by, children. For children of school age suffering from persistent infections, give a course of three or four daily for six weeks.

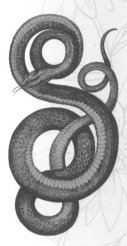

ABOVE *The Native Americans used echinacea to treat snakebites.*

Echinacea was originally a popular and effective snake bite remedy. Tradition has it that this use was discovered from watching snakes that had been bitten by other snakes.

The herb became very popular as a treatment for infections during the 19th century when it was successfully used to treat even life-threatening conditions.

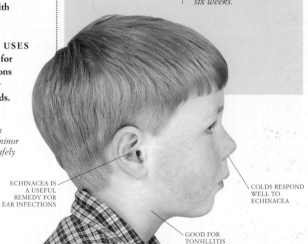

ECHINACEA IS A USEFUL REMEDY FOR EAR INFECTIONS

COLDS RESPOND WELL TO ECHINACEA

GOOD FOR TONSILLITIS

CHEMICAL CONSTITUENTS

Essential oil, resin, echinacosides, polysaccharides, including inulin.

GINSENG GRANULES

Siberian ginseng

ELEUTHROCOCCUS SENTICOSUS

The ginseng root has long been prized as one of nature's greatest cures for loss of sex drive and general debility. It has also become popular as one of the best remedies for helping people to deal with the stresses and strains of modern life.

General description

A thorny shrub from mountain woods in northeast Asia, with flowers and fruit resembling those of ivy. The roots and rhizomes (creeping roots) are used. It is sometimes called eleuthro.

Actions and character

Adaptogen (helps the body deal with stress), immune system tonic, nerve tonic, adrenal restorative.

PROFESSIONAL USES

Immune deficiencies, low blood pressure, chronic infections, chronic fatigue, diabetes, cancer, adjunct during chemotherapy and radiotherapy for cancer.

DOMESTIC USES

Ginseng is added to many commercial products. There are ginseng tea mixtures, elixirs, tonics, and even cigarettes. If buying a product such as a tonic, check that it contains an effective amount of the herb.

RECIPE

Ginseng Tonic Wine or Brandy

If the ginseng root is too hard to cut, soak for a week in wine or brandy to soften, then chop into very small pieces.

• ¼ cup (1oz/28g) ginseng root, powdered or chopped
• 8 large golden raisins
• Sprig fresh rosemary or sage
• Bottle wine or brandy

Add the first three ingredients to the wine or brandy and let stand for two weeks.

Dosage: half a small wine glass daily.

CAUTION

These herbs must not be taken during pregnancy or with coffee. Do not use in heart disease except with professional advice. Continued use may raise blood pressure and cause anxiety and hyperactivity. They are best used for short periods only.

CHEMICAL CONSTITUENTS

Triterpenoid saponins, sugars, vitamins and minerals including beta-carotene and copper.

LEFT *The Siberian ginseng is a thorny shrub with ivy-like leaves and flowers.*

RELATED PLANTS

Chinese or Korean ginseng (Panax ginseng) has similar properties to the Siberian variety but is more stimulating and less suitable for self-medication. Chewing small pieces of red (steamed) ginseng is very helpful during labor, for jet lag, and in preparation for and recovery after surgery. American ginseng (Panax quinquefolius) is very rare in its home range, due to overpicking, but it is grown in China. It was among the five most important medicinal plants of the Seneca tribe, used mostly for weakness in elderly people and as an aid to childbirth. It is considered to be milder and "cooler" than the Asian root and more fitting for weakness and prostration accompanying fevers. It is also much used for persistent lung infections with fever and dry cough. Both these herbs are more suitable for elderly people, and their main traditional use has been to maintain vitality, sex drive, and general health during old age. They are expensive, however, and other herbs such as Siberian ginseng can usually be used as a substitute. In some cases however, there is no substitute and it is worth paying more.

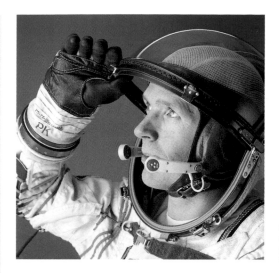

HISTORICAL NOTES

❧ Used in the Far East for thousands of years but, until recently, overshadowed by its more famous relative Chinese ginseng.

❧ Siberian ginseng became famous as the remedy that Russian astronauts used to help them cope with severe stress.

LEFT *Russian astronauts took ginseng to help them cope with stress.*

HOME USE

INTERNAL USE
• **General debility; exhaustion due to prolonged stress, weakness due to chronic disease, and for convalescence.**
• **Nervous exhaustion with loss of concentration, forgetfulness, and disordered sleep.**
• **Studying for examinations or preparing for stressful events.**
• **Impotence and low sex drive in general.**
• **Indigestion, especially from a nervous cause.**
• **Helpful in rheumatoid arthritis.**
• **Helpful in blood sugar imbalance with sudden loss of energy and craving for sweet things.**

DOSAGE

One tsp of the tincture or ½oz (15g) in decoction, three times a day.

Take ¼ –1oz (10–25g) daily as a powder or in capsules. For optimum effectiveness take a course for one month and then rest for a week before resuming.

Ginseng can also be added to other remedies for more continued use. Many tablets and capsules are available but their quality varies, so buy only from a reputable supplier.

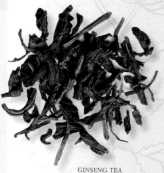

GINSENG TEA

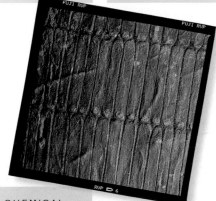

Horsetail

EQUISETUM ARVENSE AND OTHER SPECIES

DRIED HORSETAIL

Also called horsetail grass or shave grass, this strange-looking herb belongs to a primitive family of plants, often found as fossils in coal seams, which have been growing on Earth for 250 million years. Its healing powers have been known for many centuries.

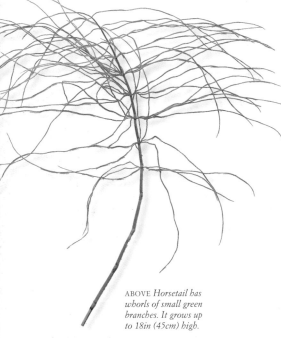

ABOVE *Horsetail has whorls of small green branches. It grows up to 18in (45cm) high.*

PROFESSIONAL USES

Connective tissue diseases, lead and other heavy metal poisoning, emphysema, and tuberculosis (as an adjunct), internal bleeding, urethritis, and osteoporosis.

DOMESTIC USES

Use as a spray or mulch on plants that have fungal infections.
Powdered herb makes a good nail polish.
At one time the plant was used for scouring pots and pans.
The young shoots can be cut in the spring and eaten as asparagus.
Horsetail ashes were used as a remedy for soaking up excess acid in the stomach.

General description

Horsetail is a perennial plant with no leaves but whorls of branches, rather like a green bottle-cleaning brush. Like the ferns to which it is related, it reproduces by means of spores that are carried in a cone at the tips of the shoots. It is a common weed on damp soil throughout the Northern Hemisphere. The whole plant is used in herbal medicine.

Actions and character

Diuretic, astringent and styptic, antifungal, strengthens bones and other connective tissues.

CHEMICAL CONSTITUENTS

Silica, zinc, selenium, flavonoids, alkaloids, saponin.

ABOVE *Horsetail is frequently found in fossil form, since the plant has been in existence for over 250 million years.*

HOME USE

INTERNAL USES
• Cystitis, chronic and acute; constant desire to pass water; cystitis with blood in the urine.
• Incontinence in elderly men with prostate problems; use for bedwetting in children.
• Water retention, especially at menopause.
• Chronic diarrhea.
• Strengthens bones, nails, and hair.
• Rheumatoid arthritis.

EXTERNAL USES
• In creams and hand and foot baths to treat fungal conditions of skin and nails.
• Compress for slow-healing wounds.
• Bath for genital irritation.

DOSAGE

Horsetail is a tough herb and must be infused for 20–30 minutes. It can be drunk cold or rewarmed. Dose: three cups a day or with other herbs.

For bedwetting, combine with St. John's wort, make an infusion and give half a cup twice daily or use the tinctures: 20–30 drops of each twice daily. Use with marshmallow and thyme for acute cystitis, with saw palmetto (Serenoa serrulata) for prostate problems, or with marigold for cellulite.

For strengthening bones and lungs and for treating arthritis, use a tincture of the fresh herb. Dose: ½ tsp (2ml) three times daily. Alternatively, simmer ¼ cup (1oz/25g) of the dried herb in 3¾ cups (900ml) water, with a teaspoon of sugar, for 3 hours in a closed vessel. Take ½ cup three times daily. These methods insure maximum extraction of the silica, which is a major healing component of the herb.

HISTORICAL NOTES

❧ Galen, writing in the second century C.E., was so impressed with the healing power of horsetail that he reported, "It will heal sinews though they be cut asunder."

❧ In 1653 Culpeper wrote in his herbal: "It is very powerful to stop bleeding either inward or outward."

❧ The herb has long been an effective remedy to stop bleeding of all kinds and also to heal bladder complaints.

❧ Recent research confirms its usefulness in arthritis, which is thought to be mostly due to its high silica content, although its other constituents also come into play.

CAUTION

Large amounts of horsetail are poisonous to cattle, but there is no evidence that the herb is toxic to humans. Blood in the urine should always be checked by a professional before beginning home treatment. Avoid large amounts and strong decoctions in pregnancy.

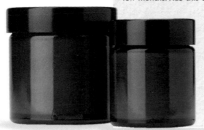

BELOW *Make a nail cream from horsetail to treat fungal infections of the nails.*

Cream for Fungal Infections of the Nail Bed

These infections result in discolored and misshapen nails. They can be very stubborn and difficult to eradicate. Once diagnosed, persist with the cream for a few months. Rub this cream well into the skin around the nails twice daily.

• 2 tsp (10ml) horsetail tincture
• 20 drops thyme essential oil
• 20 drops tea tree essential oil
• ½ tsp (2ml) St. John's wort infused oil. Olive oil makes an acceptable substitute.
• 2 tbsp (25g) emulsifying cream or any good, neutral hand cream.

❧ Add the ingredients, one by one, to the cream. ❧ Add slowly, stirring all the time.

Fennel

FOENICULUM VULGARE

FENNEL SEED

Used as a condiment since the times of the Romans and Anglo-Saxons, fennel seeds were often eaten during the Middle Ages to stave off hunger during church fasts. Fennel is especially valued in herbal medicine for its beneficial effects on the digestive system.

RIGHT *Medieval churchgoers chewed fennel seeds to prevent hunger during fasts.*

LEFT *Fennel has aromatic lime-green feathery leaves.*

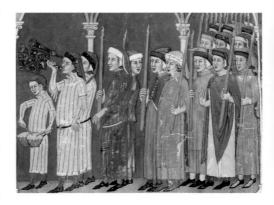

General description

Fennel is a tall, aromatic, perennial with feathery leaves and small yellow flowers borne in umbels. This wild plant of the seaside and wasteland is often grown in gardens. Cultivated forms include bronze fennel and Florence fennel (*var. dulce*), grown for its bulb-like swollen base. Parts used are the seeds (fruit), leaves, fresh stem, and root.

Actions and character.

Warming, antispasmodic, carminative, diuretic, galactogog, and antiseptic.

PROFESSIONAL USES

Fennel is used in the same manner as in the home and there are no current additional professional uses.

CHEMICAL CONSTITUENTS

Volatile oil, flavonoids including rutin, sterols.

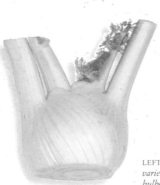

LEFT *The Florence fennel variety has a succulent bulbous root, which can be eaten raw or cooked.*

DOMESTIC USES

Fennel is used as a traditional aphrodisiac for the elderly. Fennel sauces aid digestion of fish and a fresh sprig makes an elegant garnish. The stalks from young plants may be chopped and added to salads. Powdered fennel seeds were used as a remedy against fleas in animal kennels and stables. Sweet fennel (*var. dulce*) essential oil is preferred in aromatherapy. The essential oil is used in burners to relieve asthma and wheezy coughs. A 1 percent dilution in base oil is used to massage bloated abdomens. The infused oil works as well.

HOME USE

INTERNAL USES
• Indigestion with wind and spasm. Irritable bowel syndrome.
• Stomach pain with a feeling of fullness and flatulence.
• Nausea and hiccups.
• Fennel is the best tea to take when breast-feeding as it promotes milk flow and relieves colic.
• Wind, colic, and griping in infants.
• Stubborn cough with wheezing.
• Facilitates weight loss.
• Lethargy and mild depression.
• Helpful in arthritis.
• Mouthwash for gingivitis. Also used in toothpaste.

EXTERNAL USES
• Wash or compress for sore and inflamed eyes.
• Conjunctivitis.

DOSAGE

The seeds are best used by decoction or long infusion. Crush and use half a teaspoon to a cup of boiling water. Drink three or four cups daily.

For infants with colic give 1–3 tsps (5–15ml) of the tea as required. Tea can also be made from fresh or dried leaves. This has a more delicate flavor than the seeds and will need to be made a little stronger.

For an eyewash, pour a cup of boiling water onto a teaspoon of fennel seeds and stand for 30 minutes.

Chew the seeds after rich food, to promote good and easy digestion.

Chew the seeds while fasting to diminish hunger pangs.

An inhalant for asthma can be made by crushing equal parts of fennel seeds and aniseed and burning them on a small hot plate or on a charcoal block. This is useful for children. While stroking the back, encourage the child to concentrate on inhaling the visible wisps of smoke. Panic lessens as control over breathing is re-established.

❀ Tradition has it that snakes eat fennel to clear their eyesight. A 12th-century Welsh herbal recommends it for all diseases of the eye, for persistent fevers, and for expelling poison from the body. Culpeper (1652) tells us, "The seed boiled in wine and drunk, is good for those that are bit with serpents or have eaten poisonous herbs or mushrooms."

❀ The old Greek name for fennel was "marathon," meaning "to grow thin," an allusion to its use when fasting. The famous battle of Marathon, between the Greeks and Persians, (490 B.C.E.) was fought on a field of fennel.

Old Remedy for Sciatica

The original remedy was a distillation of fennel, hawthorn, and white wine, taken with syrup of elder.

❀ Take equal parts of fennel root and hawthorn berries and make a tincture (see p. 26) with organic white wine.

Take 2 tbsp (30ml), warmed and mixed with 1 tsp (5ml) of elderberry rob (see p. 86) daily, for sciatica and persistent low back pain.

CAUTION
Avoid large amounts in pregnancy. The amounts used in cooking are safe.

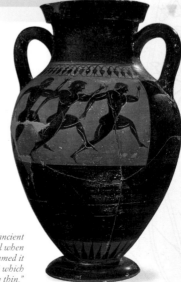

RIGHT *The ancient Greeks took fennel when fasting, they named it "marathon," which means "to grow thin."*

St. John's wort

HYPERICUM PERFORATUM

Many species of hypericum are grown in gardens but perforatum
*is the one preferred in medicine. It can be recognized by the numerous
oil glands in the leaves, which give them a "perforated" appearance
when held up to the light.*

General description

This shrubby perennial has masses of bright yellow
flowers during midsummer. It prefers dry alkaline soils
but is tolerant of a wide range of situations. Found over
most of Europe and Asia and introduced to other
countries, St. John's wort has become a troublesome
weed in North America. When the leaves are bruised,
the oil from their glands leaks out, giving rusty stains to
the plant and to the fingers when it is picked. The whole
plant has a turpentine-like odor. The tops are used,
picked in full flower.

Actions and character

Anti-inflammatory, promotes healing, analgesic, nervine,
antidepressant.

PROFESSIONAL USES

Diabetic peripheral
neuralgia; helpful in
multiple sclerosis and
Parkinson's disease.
Adjunct in radiotherapy.
With other herbs for
withdrawal from anti-
depressants, especially
from Prozac and other
serotonin re-uptake
inhibitors. For nerve
damage and depression in
A.I.D.S. Good for
interstitial cystitis.

DOMESTIC USES

There is much anecdotal
evidence of this herb's
ability to promote lucid
dreaming, a type of
practiced dreaming in
which the dreamer is able
to exercise control over
some aspects of a dream.
The flower essence is used
for fear of death, fearful
dreams, and fear from
"out of the body
experiences." It protects
those who are too open
and vulnerable, healing on
all levels and bringing
harmony.

CAUTION

St. John's wort has been called "Nature's Prozac"
but it should never be used as a substitute without
professional supervision. It is contraindicated in severe,
suicidal, and psychotic depression. Strong extracts can
cause a phototrophic rash (one which comes on in
sunshine) but this does not happen in normal
herbal use.

CHEMICAL
CONSTITUENTS

Flavonoids including the
red pigment hypericin,
volatile oil, resin, tannins.

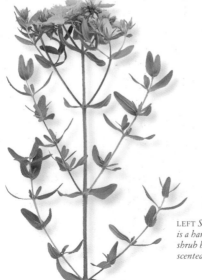

LEFT *St. John's wort
is a hardy perennial
shrub bearing lemon-
scented yellow flowers.*

HOME USE

INTERNAL USES
• Shock and hysteria.
• Mild depression.
• Menopausal depression and nervousness, menstrual pains.
• Irritable bowel.
• Stomach ulcers.
• Bed-wetting and chronic bladder inflammation.
• Two or three cups of the tea daily should help a mild depression.

EXTERNAL USES
• Puncture wounds, leg ulcers, mild burns.
• Internally and externally for pain due to nerve damage, neuralgia, sciatica, post-operative pain, and back pain.
• Internally and externally for herpes and shingles.

DOSAGE

A tincture made from the fresh plant and preparations made from it are best for internal use and as applications for cold sores, shingles and genital herpes; take ½–1 tsp (2–5ml) three times daily.

The infused oil (see the method for flowers on p. 26) is the best preparation for dressing burns, sores, and ulcers and as a massage oil for back pain and neuralgia.

Many types of tablets and drops are available and most are helpful in mild depression. Follow the instructions given.

St. John's wort combines well with vervain (Verbena officinalis) for depression, anxiety, and post-viral depression.

Combines well with horsetail (Equisetum spp) for bladder problems. For bed-wetting in children, give a cup of the tea in the early evening.

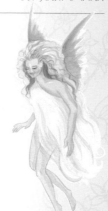

ABOVE *Don't tread on St. John's wort on your way to bed or the fairies will keep you awake, or so the legend goes.*

HISTORICAL NOTES

St. John's wort is named after St. John the Baptist, whose feast day falls on Midsummer's Day. Flowers picked before sunrise on St. John's day were said to be the most powerful, and particularly effective as a protection against witchcraft, ghosts, and evil spirits. Hypericum means "having power over apparitions."

According to legend, if someone stood on St. John's wort accidentally on the way to bed, the fairies would keep them awake all night.

Culpeper wrote that "a tincture of the flowers in spirit of wine, is commended against melancholy and madness."

RECIPE

St. John's Wort Oil

The infused oil is the best preparation for dressing burns, sores, and ulcers and as a massage oil for back pain and neuralgia.

☙ Gather the flowering tops on a dry, June morning. Put in a mortar and pestle with a small amount of vegetable oil and pound to bruise and soften. ☙ Put mixture in a clear glass jar, cover completely with oil, and shake well. ☙ Leave in the sun, shaking regularly, until the oil burns a deep red. ☙ Strain, bottle, label, and date.

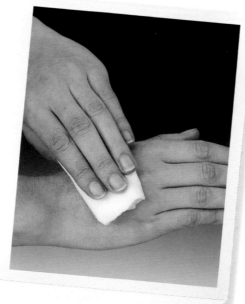

LEFT *Use the infused oil of St. John's wort to treat painful burns.*

Elecampane

INULA HELENIUM

*This tall herbaceous plant, with enormous leaves and yellow flowers
resembling double, slightly untidy sunflowers, is used to aid
convalescence and improve the spirits. It is also called scabwort,
horse dock, and elf dock, reflecting some of its traditional uses.*

ABOVE *Elecampane
has striking large
yellow flowers.*

General description

A robust perennial growing up to 6ft (2m) high,
elecampane has a woolly stem, white-veined leaves, and
large yellow flowerheads. It is a native of temperate
regions of Eurasia and has been introduced to North
America. Elecampane is easy to grow, preferring moist,
shady habitats. The rootstock, the medicinal part, is
collected in the fall.

Actions and character

Expectorant, antispasmodic, antiseptic.

PROFESSIONAL USES

Adjunct in treatment of
tuberculosis, hemoptysis,
asthma with an
overproduction of
phlegm.

DOMESTIC USES

This and related species
are used in perfume and
incense and to make
liqueurs and cordials. The
leaves of the plant are
used as a compress to
treat skin diseases in
horses and sheep.

CONVALESCENCE

*Convalescence was once an
important part of recovery
from illness, and rest homes
and convalescent homes in
rural settings were common.
People today often do not
rest properly after illness,
which makes them prone
to post-viral conditions with
exhaustion and
immune weakness.
Genuine healing and
recovery takes time. Do not
force yourself to work when
ill, and do not return to
work until you have been
symptom-free for 24 hours.*

BELOW *Skin diseases
in horses often respond
well to an elecampane
compress.*

DRIED
ELECAMPANE
FLOWERS

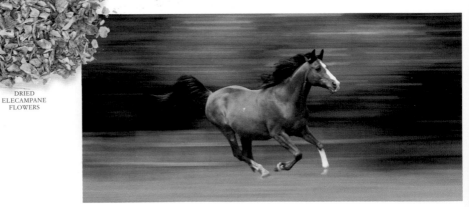

HOME USE

INTERNAL USES
• Elecampane is excellent for dry, non-productive and infected coughs, chronic bronchitis, croup, and whooping cough.
• It is also good for acute catarrhal infections.
• Lack of appetite, feeble digestion, wind, stitches and pains in the side from indigestion, from illness or old age, general weakness, convalescence, lowness of spirits.
• Mouthwash for loose teeth and gum infections.

EXTERNAL USES
• Use locally for scabs and spots.

DOSAGE

For convalescence and general debility drink three cups of the decoction a day with honey. A strong decoction will put an end to persistent dry coughs.

Traditionally, a broth was made of chicken and elecampane to aid recovery after illness.

The fresh root or a tincture made from the fresh root is best for lung and sinus infection.

Tincture dosage: ¼–1 tsp (1–5ml) three times daily for chronic conditions; double that dose for acute bronchitis and lung infections. Take in a little water or, for added benefit, in coltsfoot or elderberry syrup.

The infused oil makes an effective chest rub and a warming liniment for cold, aching joints.

The vinegar is used as a lotion for scabby, itchy skin troubles.

✂ Elecampane has a long history of use. It was known to the Romans and Ancient Greeks. In C.E. 77 Pliny reported that Julia Augustus "let no day pass without eating some of the roots of elecampane, considered to help digestion and cause mirth."

✂ Anglo-Saxon medical writers held the plant in high repute, considering it to be specific for diseases caused by mischievous elves. The candied root was sold in markets as a sweetmeat and to relieve chest complaints. It was chewed on journeys to prevent infection.

✂ In Russia, vodka flavored with elecampane is drunk for winter coughs. The Chinese use elecampane flowers (*Inula japonica*) for exactly the same purpose.

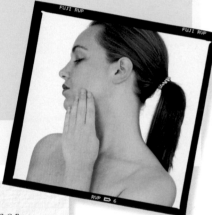

ABOVE *Use elecampane as a treatment for spots.*

RECIPE
Simon's Strengthener

This decoction is good for chronic fatigue and when convalescing from illness. Do not use in pregnancy except under the guidance of a professional herbalist. For ease of use make up several pints at a time. The tonic will keep for four or five days in a cool place. Adding a little licorice root will aid the strengthening action and improve the flavor.

✂ Take equal parts of elecampane root, crushed cinnamon bark, crushed cardamoms and lovage (*Levisticum officinalis*), or angelica (*Angelica spp*) root.
✂ Mix together well. Make a decoction using 1oz (25g) of the mixture to 2½ cups (600ml) of water.

Dosage: drink this amount over one day.

CHEMICAL CONSTITUENTS

Essential oil, bitters, saponins, mucilage, inulin.

Peppermint

MENTHA X PIPERITA

DRIED
PEPPERMINT
LEAVES

Peppermint is possibly the most popular herb in the world,
cultivated in all warm and temperate regions and often found
growing in the wild. Valuable in the kitchen, it also has a wide
range of uses in medicine as an antiseptic and analgesic.
It is one of the most effective remedies for indigestion.

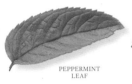

PEPPERMINT
LEAF

General description

A vigorous, fast-spreading perennial with spikes of small
lilac-pink flowers and a distinctive smell of menthol,
peppermint is a hybrid between spearmint (*Mentha
spicata*) and watermint (*Mentha aquatica*) and is quite
variable. The dark purple variety is generally regarded as
the best for medicinal purposes. Many species of mint
are used in medicine and they all have much the
same properties, with only slight differences in
emphasis between them despite noticeable
differences in taste. The common field mint
(*Mentha arvensis*) is widely used in China and
North America. Spearmint, applemint (*Mentha
rotundifolia*), and horsemint (*Mentha longifolia*)
are mostly used in cooking and to make
refreshing teas.

Actions and character

Antispasmodic, carminative, antiemetic,
diaphoretic, emmenagog. Externally
cooling and antiseptic.

CHEMICAL CONSTITUENTS

Essential oil includes
menthol, tannins,
flavonoids, bitters.

PROFESSIONAL USES

Peppermint is used in the
same manner as in the
home and there are no
additional professional uses.

DOMESTIC USES

The flower remedy is used
to promote alertness and
clarity. Fresh peppermint
may be sniffed to achieve
the same effect.
Rats dislike the smell of
peppermint.

MENTHOL

*Menthol is an ingredient of
many commercial
inhalations and liniments
but it can be irritating. It is
better to use the whole herb
or its essential oil.*

CAUTION

Do not use mints during pregnancy
(except in cooking), and avoid while
breast-feeding. It can cause digestive
upsets in babies; use catmint
(*Nepeta cataria*) instead.

LEFT *The peppermint
species has strongly
scented dark green
leaves on a purple stem.*

HOME USE

INTERNAL USES
- Spasm and colic pains; diverticulitis, colitis, and irritable bowel.
- Indigestion, flatulence and wind.
- Travel sickness, nausea, pain from gallbladder disease.
- Headaches from indigestion.
- Insomnia, especially if exacerbated by stomach tension and restlessness.
- Period pains with delayed menstruation.
- Use as a tea and inhalant for infections of the nose and sinuses.
- As a mouthwash for freshening the breath.

EXTERNAL USES
- As a compress for "hot" headaches and neuralgia.
- As a wash for hot and itchy skin conditions: the tea is cooling as it evaporates.

DOSAGE

The tea may be taken freely, although large doses may be overexciting.

Add to other herbs in teas for most digestive complaints, for example with meadowsweet (Filipendula ulmaria), and comfrey for hiatus hernia and diverticulitis. Take after rich meals to promote digestion.

For itchy skin, use the tea as a wash or add a few drops of essential oil to lotions and creams.

For inhalations (often combined with eucalyptus oil), breathe in the vapors of the tea or add a few drops of the essential oil to hot water.

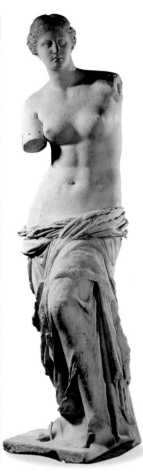

No one knows how long ago peppermint was first grown. It was first recognized as a distinct species in the 17th century but may have existed for much longer. Capsules of peppermint essential oil are recognized in orthodox medicine as a valuable antispasmodic for use in irritable bowel syndrome. In old herbals, mints are said to be aphrodisiac and to reduce breast milk. Culpeper classified mint as a herb of Venus, saying, "It stirs up venery and bodily lust."

LEFT *Because of its aphrodisiac qualities, peppermint is associated with the planet Venus, named after the Roman goddess of love.*

BELOW *Peppermint tea is an ideal remedy for fevers, nausea, colic, and indigestion.*

RECIPE
Nancy's Mint Jelly

This is a family recipe for eating with pork or lamb. It also makes a good accompaniment to nut burgers. If you have fresh rose hips, substitute them for half the weight of the apples.

- 1lb (40g) cooking apples
- Large bunch field mint (or garden mint)
- Water
- Sugar

Finely chop the mint and cut the apples into small pieces. Place in a pan and cover with water. Cook until soft. Hang them in a cheesecloth bag and let strain into a container overnight. Measure the liquid, and add 1½ cups (12oz/350g) sugar to every 2½ cups (600ml). Return to the rinsed out pan, dissolve over gentle heat; then boil rapidly to setting point. Cool, bottle, and seal.

Parsley

PETROSELINUM CRISPUM

*Parsley is probably the commonest fresh herb used in cooking.
In 1653 the herbalist Nicholas Culpeper described it as "comforting
to the stomach," and its seeds were once used with those of other
herbs to make a gripe water for children "troubled with wind
in the stomach or belly."*

DRIED PARSLEY LEAVES

General description

This low-growing biennial with finely divided leaves has
a distinctive aroma. In its second year it produces flat
umbels of small yellow flowers. The common variety has
very curly leaves but the old-fashioned flat-leaved forms
are still available, and are often preferred in European
and Indian cookery. Originally from southern Europe,
parsley is now widely cultivated in temperate climates
and often found in the wild. The leaves and occasionally
the root are used. It is easily cultivated, preferring a
shady, moist position and needing some winter
protection. The flat-leaved variety is more hardy. Parsley
seeds may take a long time to germinate – soaking the
seeds before sowing will help.

Actions and character

Antiseptic, antispasmodic,
carminative, emmenagog,
diuretic, gentle stimulant,
nourishing.

DOMESTIC USES

Chewing parsley after
eating garlic diminishes
the garlicky smell on the
breath. The herb is often
used as a garnish, but it is
a pity not to eat the
garnish since parsley is so
full of vitamins and
minerals. Parsley makes a
tasty addition to salads.
The roots of the turnip-
rooted variety (Hamburg
parsley) are eaten as a
vegetable in the same
manner as celeriac.

PROFESSIONAL USES

Compress for malignant
tumors.

RECIPE

Soupe à la Bonne Femme

This is a traditional French
recipe that is used for
strengthening women.

- 3 tbsp (45g) butter
- 6 tbsp (45g) flour
- 1 tsp (5ml) salt
- 1 medium onion, whole
- 2½ cups (600ml) milk
  or soy milk
- 1 cup (250ml) water
- 2 egg yolks
- ½ cup (120ml) cream
- 1 cup (4oz/125g) fresh
  parsley, finely chopped

Melt the butter and add
the flour, salt, onion, milk,
and water. Bring to a boil
and simmer gently for 1
hour. Remove the onion
and let cool a little. Beat
the egg yolks into the cream
and add to the soup. Heat,
without boiling. Add the
parsley before serving.

CAUTION

Do not use in
pregnancy or nephritis
(kidney disease). Parsley
seeds should not be used
internally.

RIGHT *The flat-leaved
parsley species has a
stronger flavor than the
more common curly-
leaved form.*

HOME USE

INTERNAL USES
- Rheumatism.
- Water retention, premenstrual water retention, and swollen breasts, painful urination and kidney stones.
- Painful and scanty periods. General tonic, fatigue, menopausal tiredness, and depression.
- Indigestion with wind and colicky pains.
- Eat when breast-feeding, to help replace iron and clear colic.
- Gallbladder inflammation.
- Regular use strengthens nails, hair, and skin.

EXTERNAL USES
- Compress and poultice for swollen breasts, insect bites, painful swellings in general, and sore eyes.

DOSAGE

Standard adult dose: two or three cups of the infusion of fresh or dried leaves daily.

For colic in infants, make a tea and give them a teaspoon or two.

Parsley tea makes a useful wash and compress to cool the skin, and a good lotion for weepy eczema.

Parsley and sage tea (camomile optional) is especially useful throughout the menopause.

Drink two cups a day to help maintain emotional equilibrium.

Eat parsley to freshen the breath. Constant bad breath should be investigated further.

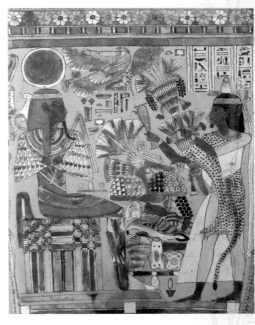

ABOVE *The Ancient Egyptians used parsley for stomach ache and bladder problems.*

CHEMICAL CONSTITUENTS

Volatile oil including apiol and myristicin, flavonoids, iron, calcium, silica, potassium, vitamins A, C, and E, folic acid. Starch and mucilage (roots).

HISTORICAL NOTES

❀ The ancient Egyptians called parsley "mountain celery" and used it for stomach pain and bladder disorders. The ancient Greeks used it for the same purposes but also commended it as a nervine for use in epilepsy. Pliny tells us that it was an old custom to crown the winners of races with a wreath of parsley, and recommends putting a few sprigs in the fishpond, to cure sickly fish.

❀ *The Physicians of Myddvai*, a 12th-century Welsh herbal, calls parsley "a generator of blood" and says it "stimulate the spirits greatly and strengthens the stomach."

BELOW *This delicious parsley soup is used by the French as a strengthening tonic for women.*

Rosemary

ROSMARINUS OFFICINALIS

DRIED
ROSEMARY
LEAVES

A warmly aromatic shrub commonly used in cooking, rosemary is also a traditional herbal remedy, highly valued for its antiseptic qualities. It has been associated with remembrance since the time of the ancient Greeks, and for hundreds of years was commonly carried at weddings and funerals as a symbol of love and happy memories.

General description

Rosemary is a woody evergreen shrub that has bluish-white flowers and narrow leaves, which are dark green above and white below. Rosemary originally came from the Mediterranean region, but it can be grown in most temperate and hot climates, preferring a sunny position in well-drained soil. Chalk soil gives the best quality. It may be trained into a hedge, but don't cut old plants back hard. The leaves and flowers are used.

LEFT *The rosemary shrub has dark green needle-like leaves.*

Actions and character

Circulatory stimulant, nerve tonic, antiseptic, carminative.

DOMESTIC USES

A weak dilution of rosemary vinegar is an excellent antiseptic and disinfectant in the sickroom.
Rosemary is included in many hair care preparations.

A few leaves under the pillow will prevent nightmares.
Flowers in linen drawers will deter moths.
A bunch of dried rosemary, picked in flower, will lift the spirits.

PROFESSIONAL USES

Chronic liver disease.

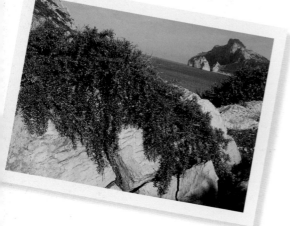

BELOW *Originally from the Mediterranean, rosemary now grows in many temperate countries.*

RECIPE

Hair and Scalp Care

Commercial rosemary shampoos and conditioners are not usually strong enough to be effective against hair loss and scalp problems. It is best to make your own.

FOR GREASY HAIR

Put two or three handfuls of fresh rosemary leaves into a jar and cover with cider vinegar. Let it stand for 10 days, then strain. Add half a cup of the vinegar to your final rinsing water when washing your hair.

FOR DRY HAIR

Use rosemary infused oil or add 1 tsp (5ml) of rosemary essential oil to 3½ fl oz (100ml) of almond oil and shake well. Rub well into the scalp, wrap with a hot towel, and leave on for 30 minutes. Wash off with a gentle shampoo.

As a general conditioner for daily use, stir 20 drops of rosemary essential oil and 10 drops of cedarwood essential oil into 3½ fl oz (100ml) of coconut oil. Use sparingly before brushing your hair.

ABOVE *Drink rosemary wine before eating to improve the appetite and aid digestion.*

BELOW *Improve the condition of your hair by using homemade rosemary preparations.*

HOME USE

INTERNAL USES

- Poor circulation, cold feet, aches and pains worse in cold weather.
- Pains in the joint that move around.
- Headaches associated with digestive troubles, including migraines.
- Depression. Poor memory. Giddiness and tendency to faint.
- Neuralgia. Transient low blood pressure.
- Hyperactivity.
- Lack of appetite, gallstones, and gallbladder inflammation.
- Hair loss and scalp problems (internally and externally).
- Good inhalant for clogged and infected sinuses and "head colds."

DOSAGE

Rosemary tea may be taken freely.

Tincture dose: 2–4 tsp (10–20ml) every day.

For general and gastric headaches, combine with camomile and take the infusion freely. For stress headaches, take with valerian.

For neuralgia, try drinking rosemary and lavender tea.

Add a few drops of rosemary and lavender essential oils to a cream for external use.

Use the infused oil as a rub for cold joints and extremities and as a chest rub.

Add 10–20 drops of the essential oil to baths for poor circulation and to improve skin tone.

Add a few sprigs to a bottle of wine and take half a wineglass before meals for poor appetite and a weak digestion.

CAUTION

Rosemary may aggravate a migraine if you take it during an attack. It is best taken as a preventive.

⁜ Rosemary is a traditional remedy for strengthening the memory and an emblem of friendship and fidelity.

⁜ Rosemary is for remembrance – sprigs were given to loved ones setting out on journeys, wreathes were worn at weddings, and a bush is often found planted in graveyards.

⁜ The distilled water of rosemary flowers was known as "Hungary water" and was a popular beauty preparation in Europe for scalp problems, to improve the skin, and also as a liniment for general aches and pains.

⁜ Posies of aromatic herbs including rosemary were carried as a protection from illness and plague. Rosemary was included in the infamous thieves' vinegar, used by thieves as a disinfectant when robbing plague victims.

CHEMICAL CONSTITUENTS

Volatile oil including borneo camphor, resin, bitters, rosmarinic acid, flavonoids.

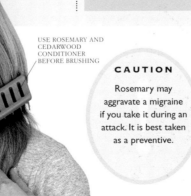

HELPS PREVENT HAIR LOSS

ROSEMARY IS A USEFUL REMEDY FOR SCALP PROBLEMS

USE ROSEMARY AND CEDARWOOD CONDITIONER BEFORE BRUSHING

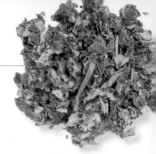

Raspberry

RUBUS IDAEUS

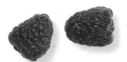

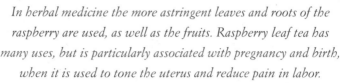

In herbal medicine the more astringent leaves and roots of the raspberry are used, as well as the fruits. Raspberry leaf tea has many uses, but is particularly associated with pregnancy and birth, when it is used to tone the uterus and reduce pain in labor.

DRIED
RASPBERRY
LEAVES

FRESH RASPBERRIES

General description

The raspberry is a shrubby, long-stemmed plant, native to the northern hemisphere and commonly cultivated for its soft, succulent fruit. The leaves and fruit are used, and sometimes the roots.

Actions and character

A gentle but firm astringent and antispasmodic.

RECIPE

Raspberry Vinegar

Raspberry vinegar is the best way of preserving the vitamin C and the therapeutic action of the fruit. It is not necessary to add sugar to the recipe.

☙ Pick sufficient raspberries to fill a large jar, cover with cider vinegar, and stand in a cool place for three or four days.
☙ Strain through a cheesecloth bag and bottle.

Dosage: take 1–2 tsp (5–10ml) in a little warm water, daily throughout the winter. This will refresh and cleanse the system, helping to prevent colds and chills.

Dilute with three parts water for use as a mouthwash or gargle. At this strength it may also be drunk freely in fevers, adding a little honey to taste. May also be used as a compress to keep you cool and comfortable.

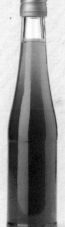

DOMESTIC USES

Blackberries (*Rubus fructicosus*) and other species of Rubus (for example, cloudberry, salmon berry) have the same properties but red raspberry leaves have the best reputation as a birthing aid. Blackberry flower remedy (from the *Rubus ursinus* species) is used to help achieve decisive action.

PROFESSIONAL USES

To prevent miscarriage.

CHEMICAL CONSTITUENTS

Tannins, polyphenols, flavonoids. Vitamin C and fruit acids (fruit only).

RASPBERRY AND BIRTH

Pregnant women are often told to drink raspberry tea, but are unsure when to do so. It should be taken during the last three months of pregnancy to tone and relax the womb, which will help to make delivery easier. To prepare for birth, drink two cups daily for the last three months of the pregnancy. Add nettles if you are anemic. During the last week add two or three cloves to each cup of tea. (Do not take cloves earlier in the pregnancy.)

For labor, make a large flask of raspberry leaf mixed with your favorite relaxing herbs and drink freely. Camomile, linden flowers (Tilia spp), and lemon balm (Melissa officinalis) will all combine extremely well with raspberry leaves.

After the birth, drink a tea with fennel seeds and raspberry leaves to assist retoning of the womb, to aid recovery, and to promote milk production and flow.

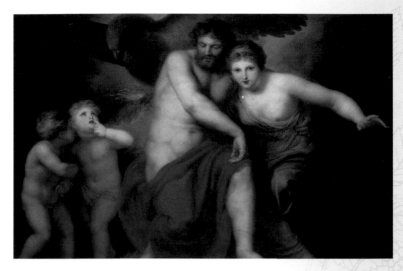

RIGHT *Raspberry's Latin
name* Rubus Idaeus
*comes from Mount Ida
in Turkey, on which
the raspberry plant
flourished. It was the
legendary hiding place of
the Greek god Zeus.*

HOME USE

INTERNAL USES
• Period pains and heavy
bleeding.
• Birth (*see left*).
• Mouth ulcers, sore
throat, chronic and
nervous diarrhea, colic.
• A decoction of the leaf
for summer diarrhea in
young children.
• Use as a mouthwash for
oral thrush.

EXTERNAL USES
• As a douche for vaginal
discharges without
infection, and for thrush.
• As a wash or compress
for inflamed eyes and sore
wounds.

DOSAGE

*Infusion: 1 tsp (5ml) to a
cup, infused for 15
minutes. Two or three
cups a day for chronic
problems.*

*Tincture: take 2–3 tsp
(10–15ml) daily. For
acute problems take more
often or use the root.*

*Tablets are available;
follow the dose given.*

*For period pains, combine
with motherwort
(Leonurus cardiaca) and
drink three cups a day
during the second half of
your cycle. Slowly chew a
fresh raspberry or
blackberry leaf to relieve
cramping pains speedily.*

*For oral thrush in babies,
fill a clean plant spray
with the tea and spray it
into their mouth.*

*Raspberry fruit and its
vinegar are used as a
remedy for sore throats
and as a cooling drink in
fevers and hot weather.*

*In China the raspberry
fruit is used for urinary
incontinence.*

HISTORICAL NOTES

The name Idaeus
comes from Mount Ida in
Turkey, which was
covered with the
raspberry plant. Greek
mythology tells how
Zeus' mother hid her son
there from his father,
Kronos, who had
threatened to kill him.

LEFT *Use
raspberry as a
wash to treat
sore and
inflamed eyes.*

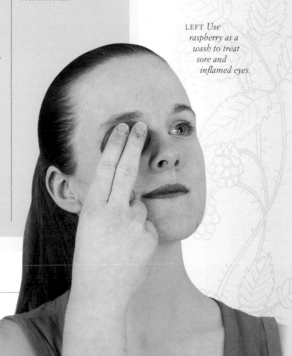

Dock

RUMEX CRISPUS

Known as a medicinal plant since ancient times, dock is traditionally used to alleviate nettle stings, thus demonstrating the cooling and healing potential of the leaves. It is its taproot, however, that is more often used in herbal preparations.

DRIED
YELLOW DOCK
ROOT

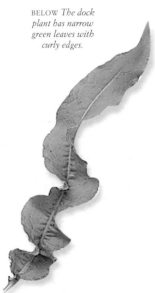

BELOW *The dock plant has narrow green leaves with curly edges.*

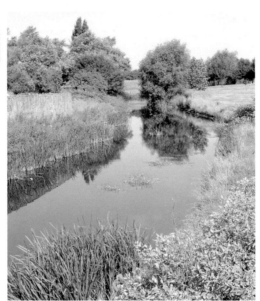

PROFESSIONAL USES

Dock is added to prescriptions to act as an alterative and promote normal function, especially for stubborn and chronic conditions.

DOMESTIC USES

Herbalists used to sprinkle iron filings around their dock plants to increase their iron content.
Dock leaves were once used as a vegetable, but they are bitter to modern tastes.
They yield a deep yellow or yellow-brown dye. Large dock leaves were used to wrap butter.
On country walks on hot summer days, put dock leaves in shoes to keep the feet cool.

ABOVE *Yellow dock can often be found growing by water.*

BELOW *Place dock leaves in your shoes to prevent feet sweating on hot days.*

General description

The yellow dock, or curled dock, is a plant of wayside, waterside, fields, and wood edges. It has narrow leaves with wavy edges and yellowish fruit. Found throughout the world, it is usually considered to be a troublesome weed in spite of its medicinal value. Many species of dock occur in different habitats. Most have similar properties, but check with local herbalists before using. Yellow dock is the one most often sold in herb stores.

Actions and character

Gentle laxative, cholagogue, alterative, tonic. Cooling.

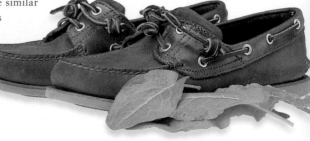

HOME USE

INTERNAL USES

• Atonic and chronic constipation, indigestion, malabsorption, poor absorption of vitamins, poor fat tolerance, sluggish liver, mild jaundice, and hot, itchy skin.

• Mild anemia.

• Skin disease, acne, pustular eczema, eczema in "hot" people, rashes that are worse in hot weather, rashes on the buttocks and psoriasis, especially when associated with digestive and liver disturbances.

• Arthritis associated with poor liver function.

• Chronically enlarged lymph nodes in children.

• Dysentery and acute diarrhea from food poisoning or infection – to expel the cause of the irritation quickly. Dock has the great virtue of clearing the bowels and then firming them up quickly afterward.

• Can be used as a mouthwash for ulcers.

EXTERNAL USES

• Ointments and compresses are used for burns, skin infections, and slow-healing wounds.

• The vinegar is used as a lotion for hot, itchy skin conditions. Diluted with an equal amount of water, it is cooling for insect bites. As a cold vinegar/water compress it is wonderfully soothing to the skin and quickly removes the heat from overexposure to the sun.

DOSAGE

Decoction: 1oz (25g) of dock root to 2½ cups (600ml) water, simmered for 20 minutes. Take ½ cup two or three times every day.

Tincture of dock root: take ½–1 tsp (2–5ml) three times daily. For chronic constipation, make a tincture combining dock with aloes and cinnamon.

The leaves can be astringent. For skin conditions the internal use of the root can be supplemented by a cooling external application of the dock leaves as a poultice, juice, or wash.

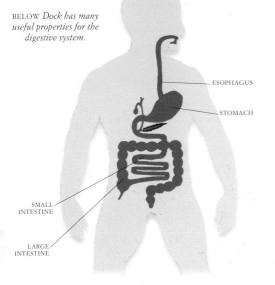

BELOW *Dock has many useful properties for the digestive system.*

ESOPHAGUS

STOMACH

SMALL INTESTINE

LARGE INTESTINE

CAUTION

When picking, do not confuse with the closely related sorrel. Sorrel possesses some of the cooling properties of dock, but their very large oxalic acid content makes them unsuitable as medicines.

CHEMICAL CONSTITUENTS

Anthraquinones, tannins, iron, vitamin C, oxalic acid.

RECIPE

Dock Vinegar

Used as a lotion, diluted with an equal amount of water for hot, itchy skin and insect bites. As a cold compress it is very soothing for skin that has been overexposed to the sun.

• 10 large dock leaves
• 1¼ cups (300ml) cider vinegar

❧ Bruise the dock leaves and cover with vinegar.
❧ Stand for two weeks.
❧ Strain and bottle.
❧ Label and date.

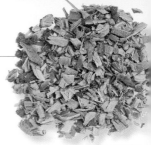

Willow

SALIX ALBA, SALIX NIGRA

DRIED WILLOW BARK

Salix alba *and* Salix nigra *are the familiar, long-leaved willows of the waterside. Willow bark is a source of salicylic acid, which is closely related to aspirin. The ability of willow bark to alleviate pain and reduce fever has been known for at least 2,000 years.*

General description

White willow is a native of Europe and was introduced to North America. Black willow is an American species often grown in parks and gardens in other countries. White willow is a tall tree with rough gray bark; the black willow is smaller, with very dark rough bark. Many species hybridize freely and are difficult to tell apart. Their medicinal value varies. The more bitter the taste, the better is the remedy. The bark, flowers, and sometimes the buds and twigs are used. Weeping willows and the golden willow are varieties of white willow.

Actions and character

Tonic, styptic, anti-inflammatory, anaphrodisiac, astringent. Cooling.

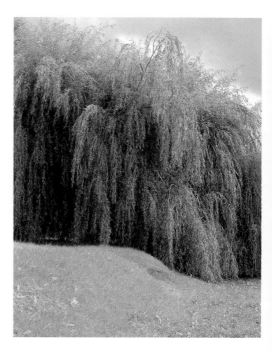

RIGHT *With its elegant drooping branches, the weeping willow is a traditional tree of mourning.*

PROFESSIONAL USES

Collagen diseases. Ovarian pain (black willow).

DOMESTIC USES

The tincture or a strong decoction is applied to the scalp for dandruff. Willow wood is light, tough, and flexible and still much used for making baskets and for fencing (although willow fences will invariably grow into a line of willow trees if the bark is left on).

CAUTION

People who are allergic to aspirin and other salicylates should avoid willow bark.

CHEMICAL CONSTITUENTS

Salicylates, tannins, flavonoids.

HOME USE

INTERNAL USES
• Inflammatory arthritis and muscle pain, gout, rheumatoid arthritis, juvenile arthritis, ankylosing spondylitis.
• Chronic diarrhea, nausea and diarrhea with digestive weakness.
• Excess sexual activity.
• Good for chronic recurrent fevers.
• Tonic after acute illness.
• With ginger for winter chills and cold winds that "stiffen the bones."

DOSAGE
Decoction: 1oz (15g) to 2½ cups (600ml) of water, simmered 15 minutes. Take ½–1 cup three times daily. For arthritic complaints, combine with celery seed (Apium graveolens) or black cohosh (Cimicifuga racemosa).

For nausea and chills, decoct equal parts of willow bark and ginger, add honey, and sip.

For headache, make a tea of willow bark and rosemary in equal parts.

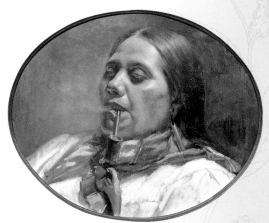

ABOVE *The Native Americans used rubbed willow bark in their smoking mixture.*

SALICYLATES
This group of chemicals related to aspirin (acetylsalicylic acid) includes salicin, which was first isolated from willow bark. Salicin proved too hard on the stomach to be a useful medicine. Aspirin itself was developed from another famous remedy for arthritis, meadowsweet (Filipendula ulmaria). Meadowsweet was originally called spiraea, *hence the name "aspirin."*

Aspirin and other so called non-steroidal anti-inflammatory drugs invariably cause stomach problems when taken in amounts large enough to control inflammatory arthritis. Herbs such as willow bark and meadowsweet do not cause this problem because their other constituents actually heal the stomach (a good example of synergy in action).

The herb wintergreen (Gaultheria spp) contains large amounts of methyl salicylate. Liniments based on wintergreen oil are effective and popular remedies for joint and muscle pain.

RECIPE

Flower Remedy
Willow flower remedy is used for rigid people who have become embittered. Willow helps them bend and move with the natural balance of the world.

• Willow flowers
• 3 tbsp (45ml) brandy
• Spring water
• 3½ fl oz (100ml) amber glass bottle

⚬ The willow flower remedy is made from the flowers of the golden willow (Salix alba var. vitellina). ⚬ In late spring, pick catkins with about 6-in (15-cm) of twig. ⚬ Pick from as many trees as possible. ⚬ Place willow and water in a pan and heat to boiling point. Simmer for 30 minutes then leave to cool. ⚬ Filter the flower water and pour 2 fl oz (50ml) into the bottle, add the brandy, label and date.

HISTORICAL NOTES

❀ At one time willow bark was the main treatment for chronic, recurrent fevers, even malaria. It was later supplanted by cinchona bark (the source of the quinine remedy).

❀ The Ancient Egyptians used willow seeds in ointments for inflamed joints and poultices for speeding the healing of broken bones. They mixed burned willow leaves with rose oil for treating scabby, inflamed conditions of the skin.

❀ Native Americans make a smoking mixture from rubbed willow bark and uva ursi (Arctostaphylos uva-ursi) leaves. This has a more pleasant smell than other herbal tobaccos.

Sage

SALVIA OFFICINALIS

DRIED SAGE LEAVES

Of all the many varieties of garden or cooking sage, red sage and the common green sage are the types preferred in medicine. It is used as a general tonic and effectively reduces perspiration, often for some days at a time.

GREEN SAGE

General description

Sage is a somewhat straggly bush with pungent, grayish, furry leaves. Originally from the Mediterranean region but now widely grown, it prefers a sunny position in well-drained soil, and is easily grown in pots and window boxes. It will stand most winters in temperate regions but may be killed in hard weather. Many varieties are available, including variegated forms. The leaves are used in herbal medicine.

Actions and character

Stimulant, astringent, antiseptic, antispasmodic, carminative, bitter tonic.

PROFESSIONAL USES

Sage is used professionally in the same manner as in the home and there are no current additional uses.

DOMESTIC USES

Strong teas, used as a rinse, will darken the hair. Use in cooking with rich, fatty meats such as pork and goose.

CHEMICAL CONSTITUENTS

Volatile oil including thujone, resin, tannins, bitters, flavonoids.

RECIPE

Sage and Onion Stuffing bake

In England the traditional Sunday roast meat was always accompanied with stuffing. Its purpose was to cut the fat of the meat, soak up juices, hide the taste and smell of bad meat, and to act as a digestive. Stuffing can be used to fill vegetables such as large tomatoes or bell peppers, or baked on its own.

- 1 small onion, sliced
- 2 tsp (10ml) sage
- 1 tsp (15ml) thyme and/or rosemary
- 1 cup bread crumbs
- 2 tsp (10ml) pine kernels or roughly chopped nuts (not peanuts)
- 2 tsp (10ml) oats
- 1 egg
- Clove garlic (optional)

☞ Mix together, stuff into meat or vegetables, or spread out a flat tray. Smear top with oil and bake for 20 minutes in a hot oven.

ABOVE Red sage has strongly flavored leaves. It may be used to treat sore throats, mouth ulcers, and gum disease.

HOME USE

INTERNAL USES
• Sore throat, mouth sores, mouth ulcers, gum disease, tonsillitis.
• Weak appetite and flatulence.
• Excessive sweating, night sweats, and menopausal hot flushes.
• Infertility.
• Painful, lumpy breasts.
• Post-viral exhaustion and the onset of viral infections.
• To prevent colds "going to the chest."
• Nervous exhaustion, anxiety, forgetfulness, depression and confusion in elderly, cold, or debilitated people.
• A good "pick me up."
• Useful for grief and after miscarriage.

EXTERNAL USES
• For cleansing infected wounds and ulcers.

CAUTION

Sage must not be used in pregnancy. Do not use while breast-feeding as it tends to dry up breast milk. The amounts used in cooking are safe. Always have breast lumps checked before treating yourself. Do not confuse sage with the sagebrushes (*Artemesia spp*) which are entirely different plants.

Sage has enjoyed a long use and high reputation as a tonic. Regular use was said to prolong life, and there are many folk sayings praising its virtues, often in alliterative poems rhyming "sage" with "a good age." In 1597 Gerard wrote: "Sage is singularly good for the head and brain, it quickeneth the senses and memory, strengtheneth the sinews, restoreth health to those that have the palsy, and taketh away shakey trembling of the members."

DOSAGE

Sage is an ingredient of many herbal toothpastes and powders. For mouth and throat problems, make a strong tea and use as a gargle or mouthwash. Add a few drops of tincture of myrrh (Commiphora molmol) to make it more effectual.

For hot flushes and sweating the cold tea is best. Dosage: ½ cup three to six times daily. The tincture is next best: take 2–4 tsp (10–20ml) daily in water.

At the onset of colds and flu take 3–4 cups of tea daily. Combines well with marigold here. For chronic complaints 2 cups of tea daily, or 3 tsp (15ml) of the tincture, will suffice.

A traditional cure for aches and pains is to chew three fresh leaves daily. A few drops of the essential oil in salt water makes a good wash for infected wounds and leg ulcers.

Sage leaves simmered for a few minutes in vinegar make a good poultice for painful or swollen joints.

BELOW *Make a poultice by simmering sage leaves for a few minutes.*

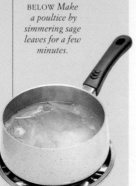

BELOW *Sage has been lauded in folk medicine for its powers to "render man immortal."*

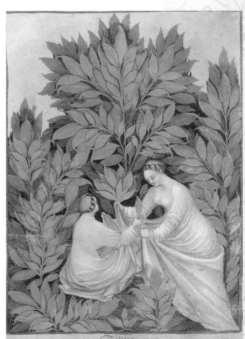

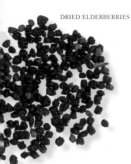
DRIED ELDERBERRIES

Elder

SAMBUCUS NIGRA, SAMBUCUS CANADENSIS

These common hedge shrubs, the European and the American elder, have so many medicinal uses that they were traditionally known as "the poor man's pharmacy," providing a cheap cure for all ills. Recent research has shown the berries to be antiviral.

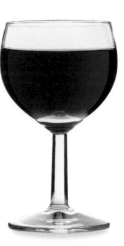

ABOVE *Elderberry wine makes a refreshing drink on hot summer days.*

General description

A small tree or shrub bearing flat masses of creamy flowers in early summer, followed by clusters of small black berries in the fall. The flowers, berries, leaves, and occasionally the bark are used.

Actions and character

Anti-inflammatory, diaphoretic, laxative, astringent, antiviral.

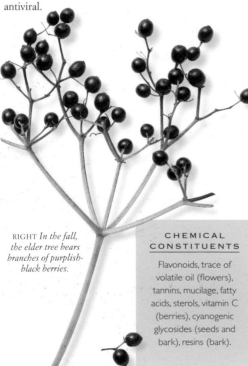

RIGHT *In the fall, the elder tree bears branches of purplish-black berries.*

DOMESTIC USES

The plant is very versatile: there are at least 50 traditional recipes using elderflowers and berries. Elderflower wine and cordial are refreshing summer drinks. Elderflower water is a gentle astringent for sore and greasy skins.
The flowers may be added to salads or made into fritters, elderflower and gooseberry jam, and water ice. The berries make an excellent port-style wine. Elderberry chutney and hedgerow jam, using elderberries, blackberries, and other hedgerow fruit make a healthy addition to the kitchen cupboard. A strong decoction of the leaves is used as a contact insecticide for greenfly infestations.

PROFESSIONAL USES

The bark is used as a laxative. Flowers are added to prescriptions for high blood pressure.

CHEMICAL CONSTITUENTS

Flavonoids, trace of volatile oil (flowers), tannins, mucilage, fatty acids, sterols, vitamin C (berries), cyanogenic glycosides (seeds and bark), resins (bark).

RECIPE

Elderberry Rob

Take elderberry rob to keep winter infections at bay. It may also be added to cough syrups, and cold and flu teas for children. They appreciate the taste, which makes many herbal teas more palatable.

• *Quantity of ripe elderberries*
• *Allspice, 1 tsp (5ml) per 2 pints (1 liter) elderberry juice*
• *Ginger (optional), ½ tsp (2ml) per 2 pints (1 liter) elderberry juice*

❧ *Strip the berries off their stalks with a fork.* ❧ *Press out the juice, using a wine press or jelly bag.* ❧ *Put into a heavy-bottomed pan, add spice(s), and reduce, over a very low heat, until the juice is the consistency of molasses.* ❧ *Bottle and store in a cool place.*

Dosage: take 1 tsp (5ml), in a cup of hot water, daily.

HOME USE

INTERNAL USES
• The flowers: for colds, sinusitis, hayfever, and as a hot infusion to promote sweating and break fevers. A gentle but effective diaphoretic, appropriate for children's fevers and for weak constitutions.
• The berries in decoction, syrup, or rob, to prevent colds and other viral infections, as a cough medicine, as a gentle laxative, and with fennel seeds for sciatica.

EXTERNAL USES
• Use as a wash for sore eyes and inflammations of the mouth.
• As a compress for twitchy eyes.
• As a cream for sore skin, chapped hands, and itchy anus.

• The leaves can be made into an ointment for painful piles and swellings and used as a compress for "hot" headaches and for painful, swollen joints.

DOSAGE

For hay fever, drink three cups a day for three months before the season. Eating the fresh flowers also gives relief from the symptoms.

Cold and flu tea: make an infusion from equal parts of elderflowers, peppermint, and yarrow and take three cups a day to prevent colds. Taken freely, this mixture will quickly resolve most fevers.

CAUTION

The flowers may be taken freely, but the berries should not be eaten raw. The flowers of other species of elder may be substituted, but their berries are often strongly laxative. Check with local herbalists before using them.

BELOW *Many folkloric tales are attached to the elder tree. It is said that you should ask permission of the tree before you cut it down or its spirit will seek revenge.*

In 1664 the diarist John Evelyn wrote of the elder, "If the medicinal properties of its leaves, bark, and berries were fully known, I cannot tell what our countryman could ail for which he might not fetch a remedy from every hedge, either for sickness, or wounds."

The tree is associated with magic. The spirit of the elder was said to be so strong, protective, and potentially vengeful that its permission should be sought before cutting.

BELOW *Try adding a little elderberry rob to your cough syrup to help ward off colds and flu.*

HELPS PREVENT VIRAL INFECTIONS

CHILDREN LIKE THE TASTE OF ELDERBERRY ROB

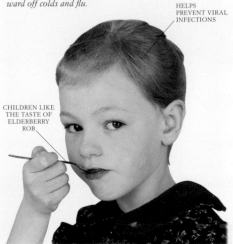

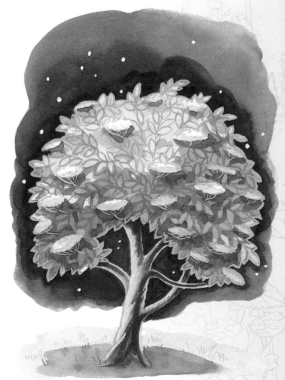

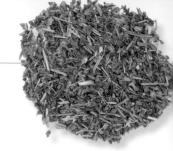

Skullcap

SCUTELLARIA LATERIFOLIA

*Also known as Virginia skullcap or helmet flower, this perennial
was used by the Native Americans to prevent spasmodic pain.
It was traditionally given to promote menstruation and to treat
the spasms brought on by rabies. The common European
skullcap (Scutellaria galericulata) has similar properties.
It is of a more creeping habit and prefers damp places.
Other species of skullcap are also used in medicine.*

LEFT *The skullcap
plant has attractive
light blue flowers in
the summer.*

General description

Virginia skullcap is a North American bushy, perennial
plant with pretty blue flowers carried in pairs, in a one-
sided spike. It is easily grown, preferring sunny, open
positions and poor soil. The whole herb is used, picked
as it comes into flower.

Actions and character

Nervine, sedative, antispasmodic.

DOMESTIC USES

The flower remedy can be
used for depression from
overwork or chronic
stress.

ABOVE *Skullcap is a
hardy perennial that
grows best in open
sunny sites.*

RECIPE

Skullcap Tea as a Simple

A simple is a remedy made
from a single herb. Many
herbs – for example,
camomile, linden,
peppermint, and fennel – are
taken as simples and this is
frequently the best way to
take them. Simples are
uncomplicated to make and
take and are always
exceptionally effective.

Use skullcap tea (see p.24)
as a simple before
examinations, interviews,
auditions, and driving tests.
Take it in stressful times
when it is important to
relax, but still be confident
and focused as it calms and
reduces tension without
causing loss of
concentration.

PROFESSIONAL USES

Epilepsy, chorea,
withdrawal from
tranquilizers and
narcotics. Helpful in
multiple sclerosis.

CHEMICAL CONSTITUENTS

Alkaloids, flavonoids,
bitters, tannins.

CHINESE SKULLCAP ROOT

Do not confuse Chinese skullcap root (Scutellaria baicalensis) with its European and U.S. relatives, with which it has little in common. It is sometimes used for insomnia and high blood pressure with excitability, but is more generally used to treat liver congestion and infections of the lung, skin, bladder, and digestive tract.

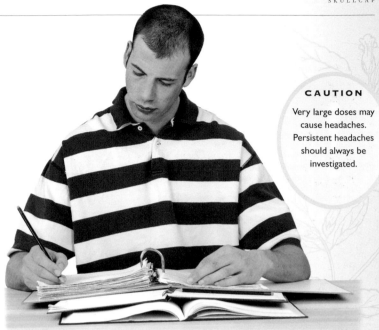

RIGHT *Drink skullcap tea before any stressful occasion such as an examination.*

CAUTION

Very large doses may cause headaches. Persistent headaches should always be investigated.

HOME USE

BRAIN

SPINAL CORD

NERVES

INTERNAL USES
• Skullcap is useful for any disorder of the nervous system – headaches, migraine, insomnia, tics, and the pain of shingles.
• Stress brought on by loss, by intensive study, or by overwork.
• Insomnia, anxiety, exam nerves.
• Exhaustion, depression, and nervousness brought on by fevers and severe acute illness or by prolonged chronic illness.

DOSAGE

Skullcap tea may be taken freely.

Tincture: 2–4 tsp (10–20ml) daily or in combinations.

Combines well with valerian for anxiety and with valerian, hops (Humulus lupulus), and passionflower (Passiflora incarnata) for insomnia, and with passiflora for insomnia due to over-excitement (suitable for children).

Take skullcap and vervain (Verbena officinalis) as a regular tea for "workaholic" tendencies, to stop burn-out and exhaustion.

HISTORICAL NOTES

❀ At one time called "mad dog skullcap" because of its use in treating rabies, in the U.S. eclectic tradition, Virginia skullcap was also recommended for fear and agitation arising from painful conditions.

❀ The European skullcap was used to treat fevers with convulsions "where the fits were more obstinate than violent," but seems not to have been a popular remedy until the introduction of the Virginia skullcap from the U.S. excited general interest in the genus.

LEFT *Skullcap is one of the main herbal remedies for disorders of the nervous system.*

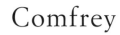

Comfrey

SYMPHYTUM OFFICINALE

The various names of this perennial plant, which is also called knitbone, bruisewort, and healing herb, refer to its long-established use in effectively mending broken bones and healing injuries.

DRIED COMFREY
LEAVES

LEFT *Comfrey has purplish-blue bell-shaped flowers from late spring.*

General description

Comfrey has large, furry leaves and drooping spikes of blue or purple flowers. Easy to grow, it prefers moist, shaded positions. Use the "officinale" species for teas rather than garden varieties. The flowering tops, leaf, and root of this wild plant are all used in herbal medicine.

Actions and character

Demulcent, emollient. Helps to promote the healing of damaged tissue.

CAUTION

Make sure that wounds are clean and free from infection before treatment with comfrey. Thorough washing with salt water or marigold tea will insure this. Smear olive oil on the skin first to prevent the fresh leaf irritating when used as a compress.

CHEMICAL CONSTITUENTS

Tannins, mucilage, allantoin, pyrrolizidine alkaloids. The allantoin promotes new cell growth in skin, bones, cartilage, and connective tissue.

DOMESTIC USES

Because it is very high in nitrogen, comfrey is commonly used as a garden mulch.

PROFESSIONAL USES

Cancerous sores, bone disease, pleurisy, and as an adjunct in tuberculosis.

RECIPE

Comfrey Liniment

This is good for muscular aches and pains, pain from old injuries and osteoarthritis.

- 1 part comfrey tincture
- 1 part "hot oil" (see Cayenne, p. 52)
- 3 drops each of rosemary and clove essential oil.

* Add essential oil at a ratio of 6 drops to 5 tsp (25ml) of the above mixture.

* To use, shake well and rub in vigorously twice daily.

LEFT *Use a pestle and mortar to mash the fresh root of the comfrey plant and apply to the area around broken bones.*

HOME USE

EXTERNAL USES
• Use a compress, cream, or ointment for sprains, torn cartilage, torn ligaments, small hernias, broken bones, osteoarthritis, aches and pains from old injuries, cuts, bruises, bleeding piles, leg ulcers, pressure sores, and mastitis.
• The mashed, fresh root will set hard and can be used on broken small bones in the same way as plaster of Paris.
• Creams, ointments, and infused oil will prevent stretch marks, if rubbed onto the abdomen during the last few months of pregnancy. They will reduce acne scarring; most scars will improve to some extent.
• Helps keep the skin smooth and wrinkle free.

INTERNAL USES
• Take the herb tea or tincture for hiatus hernia, stomach ulcers, colitis, diverticulitis, and arthritis.
• Use tea, tincture, or syrup for stubborn, dry coughs.

DOSAGE

For teas, use ½ cup (1oz/25g) of herbs to 2½ cups (600ml) water; infuse for 15 minutes. For maximum soothing, leave overnight and strain off in the morning. Drink three or four cups daily.

For hiatus hernias and stomach ulcers, combine with camomile and meadowsweet

(Filipendula ulmaria), which lowers acidity. For diverticulitis, use with meadowsweet and peppermint.

For small hernias, massage gently with warm castor oil and then apply a compress. Large hernias should be seen by a professional.

TOXICITY

Some plants containing pyrrolizidine alkaloids have been shown to cause liver damage when eaten in large amounts. There has been much debate about the possible liver damage from comfrey use and the herb has been banned for medical use in some countries. There is no evidence, however, that comfrey is toxic in normal use, and current advice is that leaf tea and tincture are safe to take internally. It is not advisable to take the root internally or to eat the plant as a food. The root may be used externally. If in doubt insure that you consult a professional herbalist.

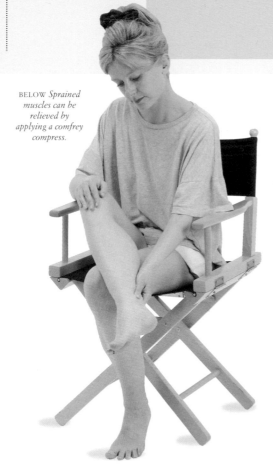

BELOW *Sprained muscles can be relieved by applying a comfrey compress.*

HISTORICAL NOTES

✀ Gerard wrote in 1597 that "the slimie substance of the roote made in a posset of ale, and given to drinke against the paine in the back, gotten by any violent motion, as wrestling, or overmuch use of women, doth in fower or five daies perfectly cure the same."

✀ In 1653 Culpeper wrote, "It is good applied to women's breasts that grow sore by the abundance of milk coming into them: as also to reprieve the overmuch bleeding of the hemorroids to cool the inflammation of the parts thereabouts, and to give ease of the pain."

Dandelion

TARAXACUM OFFICINALIS

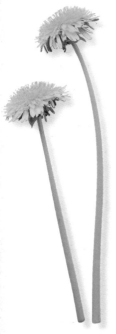

Culpeper extolled the virtues of this familiar perennial plant. Dandelion is an excellent diuretic and useful for liver disorders. Another name is cankerwort, which refers to its ability to remove toxins from the body.

DRIED DANDELION LEAVES

General description

This common wild flower, the scourge of lawn growers, is found in most parts of the world. It is distinguished by its cheerful yellow flowers, its deeply toothed leaves, and its long white taproot. The leaves, roots, and flowers are used medicinally. Dandelion has many close relatives including Chinese Dandelion (*Taraxacum mongolicum*), which has much the same properties.

ABOVE *The dandelion plant has bright yellow daisy-like flowers that close at night or in bad weather.*

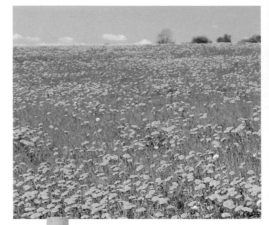

Actions and character

Liver tonic, cholagogue, diuretic, gentle laxative, detoxifier.

ABOVE *Dandelion grows prolifically in the wild, and can be found all over the world.*

RECIPE

Traditional Dandelion Wine

This wine is a clearing, slightly diuretic liver tonic and aperitif.

- 8½ pints (4 liters) boiling water
- 4 pints (2 liters) dandelion flowers, remove any green parts
- 3lb (1.5kg) sugar
- ⅓ cup (4oz/125g) raisins
- A little ginger
- The rind of a lemon
- Yeast and a small piece of toast

Pour the water on the flowers, stir, cover, and stand for three days. Strain. Add the other ingredients to the strained liquor, bring to the boil, stir well and allow to cool to blood heat. Add the yeast, spread on the toast. Cover and stand for a few days to ferment. Strain and transfer to a container. The wine will be ready in two months.

Dosage: the therapeutic dose is one small wine glass 2 tbsp (1oz/30ml), twice a day before meals.

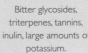

CHEMICAL CONSTITUENTS

Bitter glycosides, triterpenes, tannins, inulin, large amounts of potassium.

LEFT *Drink a daily glass of dandelion wine as a liver tonic and aperitif.*

HOME USE

INTERNAL USES
• The root is the most beneficial part for the liver. Use for liver disorders, gallbladder inflammation, mild jaundice, indigestion, chronic constipation, and constipation in pregnancy.
• The leaf is an effective diuretic. Use as a remedy for water retention, kidney stones and gravel, bed-wetting (take in the morning), and with other herbs for cystitis.
• The whole plant, by reason of its beneficial effects on the kidney and liver, is used to detoxify the body from chemicals, allergens, drugs, and anesthetics.

• The same action makes the herb valuable for chronic aches and pains, rheumatism, arthritis, and skin diseases.

EXTERNAL USE
• The milky sap from the fresh flower stalks, applied often, will clear warts.

RIGHT *A dandelion infusion is an excellent remedy for bloating caused by menstrual periods.*

DOSAGE
Dandelion may be taken freely.

For water retention, drink several cups of the infusion or decoction every day.

Concentrated forms called fluid extracts are available in specialist shops. Take 4–6 tsp (20–30ml) daily.

An infusion of the leaf with an equal amount of sage is useful for bloating during and before menstruation.

Dandelion is often combined with burdock (see pp. 44–45) for stubborn skin diseases and arthritis.

CAUTION
Large amounts of dandelion coffee can cause dull headaches in some people.

see pp. 44–45

HISTORICAL NOTES
✂ Old herbals refer to dandelion as a type of endive and recommend eating the leaves in spring "to cleanse the blood."

✂ The remedy was considered to be cooling and beneficial to people suffering from insomnia as a result of fever.

PROFESSIONAL USES
Edema and pulmonary edema from heart failure, diabetes, hepatitis.

DOMESTIC USES
The leaves are excellent in salads, and special salad varieties are available from some herb growers. The dried roots can be roasted in a low oven to make dandelion "coffee." This makes a passable substitute for coffee, especially when mixed with chicory root, and protects the liver from damage caused by coffee drinking. The flowers make excellent wine. Dandelion and burdock is a traditional soft drink. As with other soft drinks, avoid large amounts of sugar. The flower essence is used to release emotional tension held in the muscles. An infused oil of dandelion flowers is useful in massage for the same purpose.

Thyme

THYMUS VULGARIS

DRIED THYME
LEAVES

This is the common thyme of the herb garden, much used in cooking. There are many other varieties of garden thyme, mostly derived from the many different species of wild thyme. They all share the general properties of common thyme but also have their own strengths and character.

General description

Thyme is a small-leaved, creeping, aromatic plant, native to the Mediterranean region but now grown all over the world. It prefers a sunny position in well-drained soil. Either the leaves or the whole herb are used.

ABOVE *Garden thyme has aromatic leaves and tiny pinkish flowers that grow on a woody stem.*

PROFESSIONAL USES

Pneumonia, asthma with sticky phlegm. Salpingitis.

Actions and character

Antiseptic, antifungal, expectorant, antispasmodic, bronchial dilator, carminative, astringent.

DOMESTIC USES

Thyme vinegar, made by steeping a handful of fresh thyme in 2½ cups (600ml) of cider vinegar, is a useful household antiseptic and lavatory cleaner.
Take thyme honey and lemon juice for sore throats and colds.
Thyme rubbed with mullein (*Verbascum spp*) or coltsfoot (*Tussilago farfara*) makes a pleasant herbal tobacco, an agreeable alternative to cigarette smoking.
Potatoes stored with thyme keep well. Research has demonstrated that thyme works just as well as chemical antifungals in vegetable storage.
The smell of fresh thyme clears the head and is said to give courage. An inhalant of thyme oil is useful before examinations.

CHEMICAL CONSTITUENTS

Volatile oil including thymol, tannins, bitter principles, flavonoids.

RECIPE

Cough Syrup

This mixture makes a relaxing expectorant.

- 6 tsp (30ml) camomile flowers
- 4 tsp (20ml) thyme
- 2 tsp (10ml) sage
- 2 tsp (10ml) marigold flowers
- 1 clove garlic (optional)
- 2 pints (1 liter) water.
- 1¼ cups (1lb/454g) honey

☙ Add the herbs to the water and simmer in a covered vessel for 15 minutes. ☙ Strain. ☙ Return the liquid to the heat and reduce very slowly to ¾ cup (200ml). ☙ Add the honey and mix together well.

Dosage: adults, 2 tsps 4–6 times day; children, 1 tsp 4–6 times daily.

THYME IS A GOOD REMEDY FOR SORE THROATS

HELPS CHESTY COUGHS

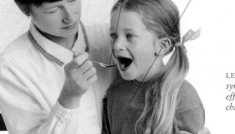

LEFT *Thyme cough syrup is a safe and effective remedy for childhood colds.*

HOME USE

INTERNAL USES
• Thyme is perhaps the best general antiseptic herb for sore throats, gum disease, infections of the digestive tract, and intestinal worms.
• Coughs, chesty colds, spasmodic and irritable coughs; considered specific for whooping cough and dry coughs.
• Cystitis and bed-wetting in children.
• Weak digestion, "liverishness," wind, and colicky pains.

EXTERNAL USES
• Athlete's foot and other fungal infections.
• Thrush.

DOSAGE

Infusions: 1 tsp (5ml) to a cup of boiling water. Drink three cups a day, more for acute infections. Inhale the vapor deeply for maximum benefit. Add a little honey for coughs and sore throats.

Use the infusion for a mouthwash or gargle, or dilute 1 tsp of tincture in ½ cup of water.

Thyme vinegar, diluted 1 to 3 with water, can be used as a douche for vaginal infections and thrush, as a wash for penile thrush, and also as a gargle.

Thyme infused oil or diluted thyme essential oil (50 drops in 3 tbsp [45ml] of olive oil) makes an effective nighttime chest rub for spasmodic coughs and lung infections and a useful liniment for arthritis and rheumatism. A few drops of the essential oil in hot water or an oil burner makes a good inhalant.

Make a talcum powder for athlete's foot by mixing 1 tsp (5ml) of thyme oil in ¼ cup (100g) of baby talcum powder or cornstarch.

❀ The antiseptic virtues of thyme have been known since ancient times. The word "thyme" means fumigation. Culpeper recommends wild thyme (*Thymus serpyllum*) for nervous disorders, headache, giddiness, and "that troublesome complaint the nightmare." He describes garden thyme as a "strengthener of the lungs" that "purges the body of phlegm."

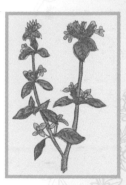

THYME

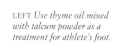

LEFT *Use thyme oil mixed with talcum powder as a treatment for athlete's foot.*

CAUTION

Avoid large amounts in pregnancy, although the amounts used in cooking are perfectly safe. Wild thyme has more of a reputation as an emmenagogue and should not be taken in pregnancy.

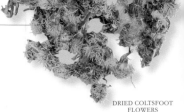

Coltsfoot

TUSSILAGO FARFARA

DRIED COLTSFOOT
FLOWERS

The scientific name for coltsfoot, Tussilago, *comes from the Greek word* tussis, *which means "a cough," reflecting this plant's time-honored use as a cough remedy. In many countries it is still a major treatment for respiratory problems generally.*

General description

Coltsfoot is a creeping, low-growing perennial that prefers heavy soils. Its flowers resemble those of the dandelion but with a central, yellow disk. This is one of the first flowers of spring and the flowers appear even before the furry, heart-shaped leaves. The leaves or the flowers with their stalks are used.

Actions and character

Demulcent, expectorant, relaxes bronchi, anti-inflammatory.

ABOVE *The leaves of the coltsfoot plant, which are very rich in zinc, are used as a remedy for coughs.*

PROFESSIONAL USES

Most chest and lung problems. As a base for smoke inhalations with other herbs, to relax the chest and restore regular breathing during asthmatic episodes, especially at night.

DOMESTIC USES

The leaf stalks are pickled in Japan and eaten as a relish. The flower stalks may be eaten and make a tasty and unusual addition to stir-fried vegetables.

CHEMICAL CONSTITUENTS

Mucilage, bitters, saponins, zinc, pyrrolizidine alkaloids.

BELOW *Herbal "tobacco" made from coltsfoot and other herbs is used to treat chronic lung complaints.*

CAUTION

The presence of pyrrolizidine alkaloids in coltsfoot has raised worries about possible liver damage, but there is no evidence that taking coltsfoot medicinally is harmful. Nevertheless, avoid eating large amounts of the plant if you are pregnant or breast-feeding (see also Comfrey, pp. 90–91).

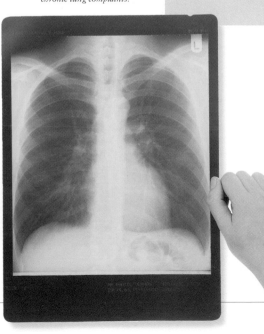

HOME USE

INTERNAL USES

• Dry, persistent, and wheezy coughs; specific for chronic bronchitis.
• For infected and productive coughs, add 2 tsp (10ml) of garlic honey, or make an infusion with coltsfoot and thyme.

EXTERNAL USES

• Herbal "tobacco" based on coltsfoot is traditionally smoked by those wishing to give up smoking, and for chronic lung problems.
• Use locally for slowly healing wounds and in a cream for broken veins.

DOSAGE

For the maximum soothing effect, soak 1oz (25g) in 2½ cups (600ml) of water overnight. Strain and drink throughout the whole day.

For chronic "smokers cough," an ordinary decoction or syrup taken three times daily will usually suffice.

SIMILAR PLANTS

MULLEIN

Mullein (Verbascum thaspus) is a beautiful wildflower with a tall, thick spike of yellow flowers found in most temperate regions of the world. It is the second most popular herb in herbal tobacco and a significant lung tonic in its own right. Mullein syrup and tea are particularly helpful for asthma and bronchitis with thick, sticky mucus, when it is a more useful remedy than coltsfoot. A traditional Irish remedy for tuberculosis was made by boiling the fresh leaves in milk and adding honey. An infused oil made from the flowers is used as ear drops for chronic earache and itchy ears.

HISTORICAL NOTES

❀ Coltsfoot was at one time used for tuberculosis and was said to have been helpful in silicosis. The ancient Roman Pliny in his *Natural History*, written in the 1st century, recommends burning coltsfoot leaves and inhaling the smoke for coughs. The 17th century herbalist Culpeper recommends coltsfoot and elderflower for fevers and the syrup for "a bad, dry cough, or wheezing and shortness of breath."

❀ In the English countryside, the soft, downy underside of the coltsfoot leaf was once scraped off and used as tinder to start fires.

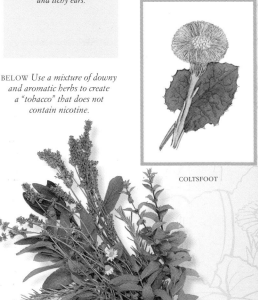

COLTSFOOT

RECIPE

Herbal "Tobacco"

Herbal "tobacco" contains no nicotine. The herbal "tobacco" can be burned on a charcoal block and the smoke inhaled, rolled in paper, or smoked in a pipe. Several herbs are used as the basis for herbal "tobaccos." They include coltsfoot, sage, and mullein. These are all downy herbs beneficial to the lungs. Downy herbs are chosen because they burn evenly and easily. A good "tobacco" includes at least half of one of these herbs, or a mixture of them. The other ingredients are usually aromatic herbs such as camomile, thyme, mint, lavender, and rosemary, or calming herbs such as skullcap. The herbs should be cut small, mixed together thoroughly and then rubbed between the hands until they are well blended. For a smoother smoke, dissolve 1 tbsp (5ml) of honey in a little water and stir into the herbs. Spread the mixture out on a tray until dry enough to burn evenly. This will take around a day or two. Store in airtight containers.

BELOW *Use a mixture of downy and aromatic herbs to create a "tobacco" that does not contain nicotine.*

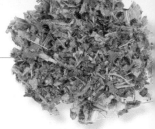

Nettle

URTICA DIOICA

DRIED NETTLE LEAVES

The common stinging nettle is a perennial plant found all over the world. It has always been highly valued as a remedy for many different ailments, as well as for its high nutritional content – it is rich in iron – and for "cleansing the blood" in spring.

General description

The young leaves, roots, and seeds are used. The common stinging nettle has a square, bristly stem up to 7ft (2m) high and deeply serrated, with pointed leaves that are downy underneath. This plant will grow almost anywhere, but prefers well-dug, rich soil such as in compost heaps and the edges of farmland.

ABOVE *Nettles are rich in iron, which is absorbed from the soil. The plant should be harvested when flowering.*

Actions and character

Blood tonic, styptic, mild diuretic, anti-allergic, nutritive.

PROFESSIONAL USES

Nettles are used with other herbs to treat kidney disease and diabetes. The tea relieves itching in Hodgkin's disease. The roots are used with saw palmetto (*Serenoa serrulata*) for benign prostatic hypertrophy.

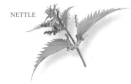

NETTLE

DOMESTIC USES

This is the food plant of many useful insects and caterpillars. It also makes an excellent mulch, and should be grown in all gardens with sufficient space. Nettle fiber can be woven into cloth. The leaves yield a rich, green dye and the roots make a yellow dye. The annual nettle (*Urtica urens*) is used in homeopathy for nettle rash and burning sensations. The young top leaves can be collected throughout the year, steamed, and eaten like spinach or made into a soup. Cooked nettles do not sting.

SPRING CLEANING

*Spring is a time of regeneration: the sap rises, new energy sloughs off winter, and the sun returns. Traditional spring-cleaning rituals included putting away winter's clothes, steaming or birching the skin, and fresh green food and drink. Young nettles and other herbs were customarily eaten during the spring to cleanse the skin, lift the spirits, and clear the heaviness and lethargy left behind by winter. As we spring clean the house, so we should spring clean the body. A good herbal cleanser, useful at any time of the year for persistent spots and rashes and for the heaviness of over-indulgence, is a tea made from equal parts of nettles and cleavers (*Galium aparine*). Drink three cups a day for several weeks.*

CHEMICAL CONSTITUENTS

Large amounts of minerals and vitamins including iron, potassium, calcium, silica, and vitamin C. The stinging hairs contain formic acid and histamine.

CAUTION

Take care when picking nettles; their bristly hairs contain histamine and formic acid, which sting. Very large doses may cause a burning itch in some people. Do not eat mature plants uncooked as they can cause liver damage.

HOME USE

INTERNAL USES
• Take fresh juice or an infusion for iron-deficiency anemia, and for mineral deficiency with lethargy and pallor.
• Drink the tea to relieve heavy menstrual bleeding.
• Nettle juice or tea is a useful drink during pregnancy and while breast-feeding.
• Juice or tea is helpful in gout and rheumatoid arthritis.
• Take an infusion for nettle rash, allergic reactions to shellfish, strawberries, etc., and for nervous eczema.
• Nettle seeds are helpful in asthma.

DOSAGE

For most purposes, three or four cups of the tea a day will suffice. For nettle rash use several cups a day for three or four days.

For severe deficiencies use 4–6 tsp (20–30ml) of the juice or a bowl of nettle soup, daily, or take the iron tonic.

This is a very useful herb for those of a lethargic disposition.

RIGHT *Drink three or four cups of nettle tea daily as a treatment for nettle rash.*

EXTERNAL USES
• For stiffness and osteoarthritis, rub the affected joint with fresh nettle leaves.
• For nose bleeds, sniff fresh nettle juice through the nostrils.
• Make a compress as a treatment for burns.
• Infused oil is useful for inflamed psoriasis.
• Use tea or tincture as a wash for falling hair and dry scalp.

HISTORICAL NOTES

❀ Various species of nettle found around the world have been used for medicine and cloth-making since the beginning of recorded time. Nettles from warmer climates tend to be more virulent.

❀ Roman soldiers were said to have brought their nettle (*Urtica pilulifera*) north with them and used it to rub their skin to keep out the cold. This nettle can still be found growing around Roman ruins in northern Europe.

BELOW *The Romans rubbed nettles on their skin to keep out the cold.*

RECIPE
Iron Tonic

This tonic is especially useful during pregnancy.

- *2 handfuls dried nettle leaves*
- *1 handful dried unsulfered apricots*
- *8 organic almonds (optional)*
- *Peel from 1 large, bitter orange, preferably unwaxed*
- *1 bottle red wine, preferably organic*

❦ Put the dry ingredients in a large jar and cover with the wine. ❦ Leave for two weeks. ❦ Shake from time to time. ❦ Strain into amber or green glass bottles and store in a cool place.

Dosage: 2–4 tsp (10–20 ml) twice every day.

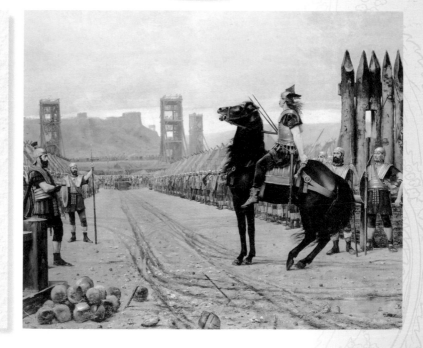

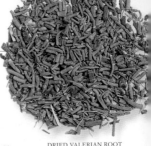

Valerian

VALERIANA OFFICINALIS

DRIED VALERIAN ROOT

*Also called fragrant valerian because of its strong smell,
valerian was used in the past to make perfume, but it is
considered too pungent for that purpose today. The root is the part
used medicinally, and it is useful for all sorts of nervous conditions
including migraine, anxiety, and insomnia.*

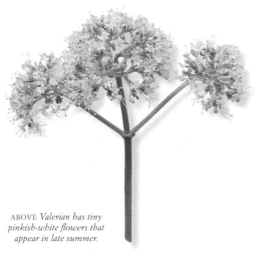

ABOVE *Valerian has tiny
pinkish-white flowers that
appear in late summer.*

PROFESSIONAL USES

High blood pressure,
epilepsy, and withdrawal
from benzodiazepines and
other drugs. Valerian is
non-addictive and makes
a good substitute for
sedative drugs.

DOMESTIC USES

The leaves may be used in
salads. Cats and rats are
very fond of valerian and
may destroy the plants.
Cats enjoy toys smeared in
the tea or tincture. It does
them no harm. At one
time rat traps were baited
with valerian.

CAUTION

The key word for valerian is anxiety.
Excessively fiery people, kept awake by over-
activity rather than anxiety, may find their symptoms
exacerbated. Large or extended doses may leave a
heavy head, so for this reason combined tablets
are preferred for general use. Valerian is
not suitable for small children.

VALERIAN LEAF

General description

Valerian has long, winged leaves with small pink or
white flowers in rounded clusters. It grows in a variety of
soils, preferring either ditches or wood edges on chalk
downland. It grows slowly but is persistent when
established. The whole plant including the root has a
strong, distinctive smell, disliked by some people. Other
species of Valeriana may be substituted, but check in a
local herb book before using. Red valerian (*Centranthus
ruber*) is a related species with different properties.

CHEMICAL CONSTITUENTS

Volatile oil including
valerianic acid and
borneol, volatile
alkaloids, resin.

Actions and character

Relaxant, sedative, carminative, antispasmodic, mildly
anodyne.

HOME USE

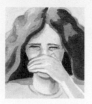 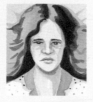 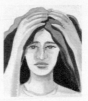

ABOVE *Valerian can be used internally for anxiety, insomnia, coughs, and migraines.*

INTERNAL USE
• Insomnia, anxiety, anxiety with depression, general irritability, irritable cough, tension headaches, migraine, panic attacks, palpitations, menstrual pain, irritable bowel, stress constipation, and intestinal cramps.
• A useful calming remedy for tension and anxiety.
• It is a strengthening nerve tonic when taken over a period of time.
• Helpful in neuralgia, vertigo, and tinnitus.
• A compress can be used for headaches.

DOSAGE

The cold decoction is best: place 1 tsp (5ml) of chopped root in a cup of water, stand overnight, and drink throughout the next day.

Tablets and compound tablets are widely available; follow the directions on the package. Valerian is also commonly combined with skullcap, hops, wild lettuce, or passionflower.

Different combinations suit different people:

For tension migraines; equal parts of valerian and feverfew tincture, 1–2 tsp (5–10ml) per day.

For irritable bowel with constipation, combine with marshmallow and dock root. For wind and colic, combine with camomile.

For irritable cough, make a syrup with valerian, thyme, and coltsfoot.

For stress, a decoction made with ½ tsp (2ml) of valerian and a few cardamoms to a cup of water, taken with honey, is a relaxing drink.

HISTORICAL NOTES

❀ Valerian was known as "heal all and set well" to the ancients. It was used to strengthen the eyesight, as a cough medicine, to heal infected wounds, and to resist the plague.

❀ The ancient Greek writers called it "phu" in allusion to its smell, and in the 16th century it was put in among bedlinen – possibly to induce restful sleep rather than to lend a pleasant smell.

❀ In more recent times, it was widely used to combat anxiety and insomnia from air raids, and was a well-known medicine until the introduction of modern tranquilizers.

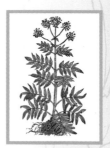

VALERIAN

RECIPE
Deep Sleep Mixture

It is natural to suffer occasional nights of insomnia, especially during times of stress, excitement, or bereavement. If it becomes a habitual or worrying problem, seek professional advice. Keep this old-fashioned remedy for occasional nights of restlessness, with light or continually broken sleep.

❧ Take equal parts of dried valerian root, hop flowers, and passionflower leaves, place in a jar, and cover with vodka (or 40% alcohol). ❧ Stand for two weeks, shaking occasionally. ❧ After this time, strain and add an equal volume of linden flower honey. ❧ Shake well and store in a dark bottle.

Dosage: 2–4 tsp (10–20ml) at bedtime.

BELOW *Historically valerian has had a wide variety of uses.*

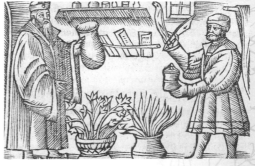

Vervain

VERBENA OFFICINALIS AND VERBENA HASTATA

DRIED VERVAIN LEAVES
AND FLOWERS

*Vervain or verbena is the only herb that was sacred
to both Celtic Druids and Anglo-Saxon shamans, who wore
it to protect themselves from evil spirits. It has great powers
as a healing herb, particularly for wounds, and also acts
as a nerve relaxant and antidepressant.*

General description

European vervain (*Verbena officinalis*)
is a Eurasian plant but is found as a
weed in many parts of the world,
including North America. It is a
medium-sized perennial with an
open habit and long spikes of small,
pale pink flowers. It is easy to grow,
preferring well-drained soils. Blue
vervain (*Verbena hastata*) is a
native of North America. It
has a more bushy habit and prefers
damper soils. The whole herb is
used, picked as it is coming into
flower. Various verbena
hybrids are grown in gardens,
but these are not used in medicine.

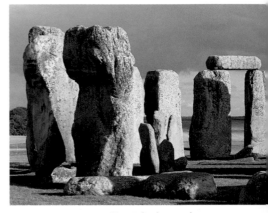

ABOVE *Vervain has been used as a
sacred plant for thousands of years.*

Actions and character

Relaxing nervine, antispasmodic,
antidepressant, diaphoretic, diuretic,
galactagog, antiseptic, bitter tonic,
general tonic.

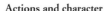

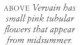

ABOVE *Vervain has
small pink tubular
flowers that appear
from midsummer.*

**CHEMICAL
CONSTITUENTS**

Alkaloids, flavonoids,
volatile oil, tannins.

R E C I P E

Vervain Flower Remedy

This remedy is for strong-
minded individuals who
believe they are always right.
Used to balance personal
will with tolerance and
understanding.

• Vervain Flowers
• 3 tbsp (45ml) brandy
• Spring water
• 3½ fl oz (100ml) clean
amber glass bottle

☙ Pour spring water into a
clean glass bowl, float
flowers on the surface and
place in direct sunlight for
3 hours. Pour 2 fl oz (50ml)
into the bottle, add brandy,
label and date.

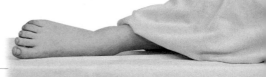

HOME USE

INTERNAL USES
• Fevers, especially those with headaches or deep, aching pains.
• Nervous exhaustion from overwork.
• Post-viral fatigue and exhaustion.
• Liverishness and indigestion, especially following infections; mild jaundice.
• Intestinal worms.
• Kidney stones and water retention.
• Asthma and hayfever with tight chest muscles.
• Promotes milk production in nursing mothers; especially useful when the new mother is anxious and stressed.
• Depression with aches and pains or digestive disturbances.
• Insomnia and restless sleep; excessive dreaming.
• Painful periods.

EXTERNAL USES
• Ointment for painful swellings, piles, and slow-healing wounds.
• Poultice or compress for headaches and muscle aches.

DOSAGE
Take the infusion freely for acute fevers; take three cups a day for exhaustion.

Tincture dose: 1– 2 tsp (5–10ml) three times daily. The fresh plant tincture is best if available.

For insomnia or nightmares take 2 tsp (10ml) at night in a little warm water.

Combines well with St. John's wort for mild depression and neuralgia, and with betony (Stachys betonica) or sage for post-viral exhaustion.

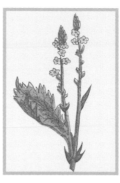

VERVAIN

PROFESSIONAL USES
Paranoia, post-natal depression, epilepsy, and convulsions. Convulsions with fever.

DOMESTIC USES
Vervain is one of the original 12 flower remedies discovered by Dr. Edward Bach.

In early times vervain was seen as a talisman with the power to drive away the devil and evil spirits. The herbalist John Gerard (1597), however, had no time for these "fables tending to witchcraft and sorcery... as honest ears abhor to hear."

Culpeper (1653) recommends vervain for "cold distempers of the womb," and describes it as a good remedy for inflamed and infected wounds including ulcers and fistulas.

The Grete Herbal of 1526 gives this recipe: "To make folk merry at the table, take four leaves and four roots of vervain in wine and sprinkle the wine all around the house."

CAUTION
Do not use in pregnancy. Large doses may cause vomiting.

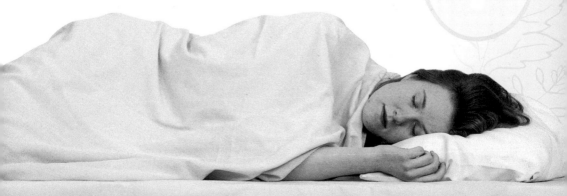

BELOW *If you suffer from insomnia, try taking vervain for a deep, relaxing sleep.*

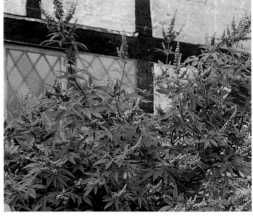

Agnus castus

VITEX AGNUS-CASTUS

DRIED AGNUS
CASTUS BERRIES

This herb, also called the chasteberry or chaste tree, has been much researched in Germany and its fruits have been shown to have a regulating effect on the pituitary gland, tending to promote production of the hormones progesterone and prolactin.

General description

The chaste-tree is an elegant shrub native to the eastern Mediterranean and western Asia, and naturalized in the southeastern United States. It can be grown in more temperate climates if protected from the worst frosts. The berries, which have a slightly bitter and peppery taste, are the part used medicinally.

Actions and character

Hormone regulator, tonic for the nervous system.

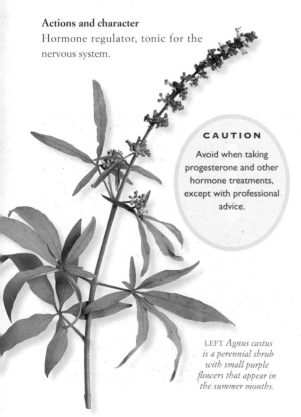

ABOVE *Originally from the Mediterranean and western Asia, agnus castus can also be grown in temperate regions.*

CAUTION

Avoid when taking progesterone and other hormone treatments, except with professional advice.

PROFESSIONAL USES

Heavy menstrual bleeding and bleeding between periods. Endometriosis. Pituitary disorders.

CHEMICAL CONSTITUENTS

Volatile oil, iridoid glycosides, bitters, oils, alkaloids.

DOMESTIC USES

Black pepper was once a rare and expensive condiment. The dried fruit of agnus castus was powdered or ground and used on food as a substitute for, or in combination with, black pepper. It has an interesting slightly peppery taste. Try it!

LEFT *Agnus castus is a perennial shrub with small purple flowers that appear in the summer months.*

HOME USE

INTERNAL USES
- Premenstrual syndrome, including mood swings, depression, water retention, and breast pain.
- Menopausal hot flushes and mood swings.
- Lack of periods and infertility due to hormonal imbalance. Irregular menstrual cycle. To re-establish regular periods after birth.
- For withdrawing from the contraceptive pill.
- To promote milk flow in nursing mothers.
- Nervous excitability.
- Weakness and headaches that are due to nervous tension.
- Excessive sex drive in men due to high testosterone levels.

DOSAGE

For premenstrual syndrome (P.M.S.): take the decoction, one cup daily, or the tincture, 20–30 drops daily. Most effective taken first thing in the morning. Tablets are available; take according to directions.

For menopausal problems combine with sage, motherwort (Leonurus cardiaca), and St. John's wort. Take two or three cups a day of the combined decoction or 3 tsps (15ml) a day of the combined tincture.

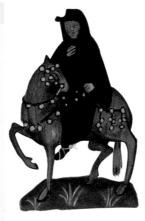

ABOVE *Agnus castus was traditionally taken by monks as it was reputed to reduce their sexual urge.*

BELOW *Nursing mothers used vervain to promote lactation in the 17th century.*

HISTORICAL NOTES

Agnus castus was traditionally used to insure chastity in monks, hence its common alternative names and the old name monk's pepper.

It was also used to promote milk flow and for lack of periods. The English herbalist Parkinson (1629) says, "[it] procureth milke in women's breasts" and "a decoction of the herbe and seede is very good for paines of the mother, or inflammation of the parts." The "mother" was the traditional name for the womb.

In China and India, *Vitex spp* are used for nervous tension, muscle pains, and to relieve colds.

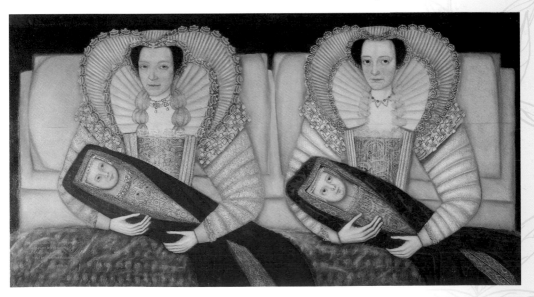

Herbalism at Home

*ALL HUMAN BEINGS are constitutionally adapted for survival. This impetus
to life, sometimes called the Vital Spirit, can be heroically strong in some people,
overcoming extremes of adversity and suffering. Herbal medicine works with this
power, and with the many protective, defensive, balancing, and healing mechanisms
of the body. The aim of herbal medicine is to help the body help itself, encouraging
and supporting the elimination of toxins and strengthening weakened tissues.*

MAINTAINING GOOD HEALTH

Good health is for everyone, not just the young, active, and able-bodied. Health is a sense of well-being, of feeling comfortable and confident in one's body, knowing that it is possible to meet everyday physical and emotional challenges with resources to spare.

When we are young, we tend to take our health for granted. A graze heals, a break mends, colds run their course, and somehow the body continues with a strong momentum toward maintaining well-being and health. As we age, however, stress takes its toll, and we may become less confident in our body's innate ability to heal itself. Pollution, the bad habits of a lifetime, and the demands of modern living, all these factors can stress the body. The health-giving properties of herbs, which have been known for many centuries, can play a vital part in our health, helping to counter the effects of stress and illness with their wonderful healing powers.

Achieving and maintaining general good health is an individual process – what is a suitable activity for one person, for example, might be an exhausting strain for another.

There are, however, a few basic requirements that we need to maintain good health:

• Good-quality and nourishing food and herbs.
• Pure clean air and water.
• Adequate warmth and shelter.
• Careful balance of work, rest, and play.
• A sense of purpose.
• Self-worth – a feeling of belonging and contributing.

Your emotional and spiritual well-being is just as important as your physical state when you assess your level of health.

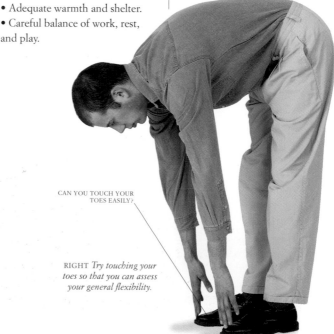

CAN YOU TOUCH YOUR
TOES EASILY?

RIGHT *Try touching your
toes so that you can assess
your general flexibility.*

YOUR ANNUAL CHECK UP

To maintain optimum health, you need to develop a lifestyle that encourages health and avoids situations that "make you sick," either physically or mentally. An annual physical check-up that you can do yourself at home will help you to monitor your general health. It will allow you to notice any signs of illness, and indicate areas that may need support, a change of routine, or medical treatment. Examine the breasts or testes. Look at your skin, noting its color and any warts or blemishes. They should be unchanged from previous years.

• Check your weight.

• Check your general mobility and specific joint mobility (try to reach the top cupboards, touch your toes).

• Test your lung capacity (try blowing up a balloon).

• Exercise, to check your stamina and recovery time (run up stairs).

• Do these checks after any long illness or period of convalescence to make certain that you have regained your optimum health.

Assessing illness

Whether your illness is of long duration or sudden onset, accurate information is essential, in order to plan treatment, choose appropriate herbs, to monitor progress, and to know when to call for professional help. With children in particular, it is important to respond to the first sign of discomfort.

Ask the following questions and note down the answers.

• What is wrong?

• If there is pain, what kind of pain (for example, stabbing, dragging, aching, numb, sharp) is it?

• Is the pain constant or intermittent?

• Where does it hurt?

• What size and shape is the painful area?

• When did it start?

• What makes it better and what makes it worse?

• What other symptoms do you have?

Observe any changes in your appearance, and take your temperature if appropriate. Making a list of specific symptoms such as discharge from the nose, dry eyes, and general listlessness is more useful than an overall diagnostic label such as flu.

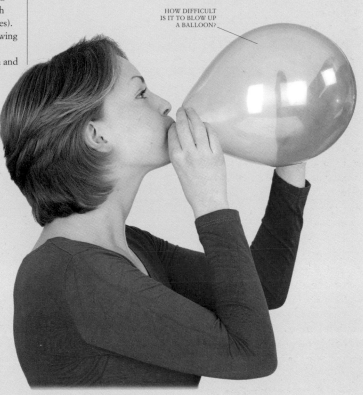

HOW DIFFICULT IS IT TO BLOW UP A BALLOON?

RIGHT *To test your lung capacity, blow up a balloon. You should be able to do it without too much effort.*

Treating Illness at Home

HOLISTIC TREATMENT *of illness is mainly common sense, and most people will intuitively consider all the factors below. But illness is a time of stress, and in responding to the distress of a loved one, it is easy to forget or overlook small matters. It is important to remain calm, and act carefully and methodically.*

ABOVE *When you are treating yourself at home, keep a note of everything you do and take.*

• Cut down on immediate stress.
• Consider your diet, rest, exercise, massage, any changes in routine.
• Decide on the best herbs and their method of application; internal or external. Think of baths, washes, lotions, gargles, douches, syrups, etc., and the minimum treatment needed to be effective.
• Plan a treatment regime, working with the body to:
a. alleviate symptoms
b. strengthen the body so that it may help itself.
• Understand the herbal strategy and know what to expect. Take the recommended dosage only.
• Keep a note of everything you do and take. Monitor the response. Make changes if necessary, or seek professional help.
• After treatment, check that health is fully regained. Take time to rest and convalesce if necessary. Plan a strengthening or convalescent regime if required.
• Make notes of observations and learn from the experience.

HOME TREATMENT CASE
STUDY ONE • AN ACUTE CASE

Richard, aged 28, with a mild fever, slight sore throat, and general nervous listlessness. Uncomfortable in own body.

TREATMENT PLAN
Reduce stress. Stop work.
Day 1: Light diet, bed rest, herbal tea x 6. Gargle with salt and sage every 4 hours.
Day 2: Light movement, herbal tea x 4, herbal bath. Gargle night and morning
Day 3: Restore diet. Light exercise. Herbal tea as preventive x 3 for rest of week.
Day 4: Back to work.

HERBAL STRATEGY
Medicinal herbal tea.
Equal parts of four herbs:
PEPPERMINT to clear head and sinuses.
ELDERFLOWER to clear and strengthen nose.
YARROW to help fever.
CAMOMILE to relax and help listless feeling.

RIGHT *A sage gargle helped to clear Richard's sore throat, and herbal baths relieved his symptoms of stress.*

Sage Gargle
An antiseptic, soothing and tonic gargle, to relieve dry sore throats.

RESULTS OF MONITORING
Day 1: Found it hard to rest; gargle most useful.
Day 2: Slept right through, till 11 am. Did not realize I was so tired and stressed. Took it easy. No temperature. Throat less sore.
Day 3: A good night's sleep. Very hungry, ate cooked breakfast. Went for walk. Plan for tomorrow.
Day 4: Recovered and back at work. Continued tea but only twice today as it is not convenient to make at work. Herbal bath: put 15 drops rosemary oil in bath (to relax, clear head, draw out impurities, improve circulation). I wish I had remembered this earlier.

OBSERVATION
What was needed was rest and recuperation. Remember to gargle at first sign. Stop work at temperature. Do not return till temperature is normal for 24 hours. Watch for signs of stress. Forget the shower and soak in a herbal bath when stressed.

HOME TREATMENT CASE
STUDY TWO • A CHRONIC CASE

William, aged 73, with hand pain and finger stiffness in the morning, getting worse. Fearful of winter and cost of heating.

TREATMENT PLAN

Reduce stress by changing diet.
Include large amounts of vegetables and greens. Reduce coffee.
Warm hand bath daily.
Herbal tea x 3 per day.
A decoction when pain is bad, internally and externally.
Warming foot bath when needed.
Follow regime for two months' trial.

HERBAL STRATEGY

Little or no coffee to reduce irritants and stimulants.

Hand bath
JUNIPER essential oil to warm and aid clearing and elimination.
CAMOMILE to relax and reduce inflammation.
5 drops of each essential oil per 2½ cups (600ml) warm water, soak for 10–20 minutes.

Medicinal herbal tea.
Equal parts:
MARIGOLD as an anti-inflammatory.
PARSLEY to help elimination (juniper may be too strong internally).
DANDELION AND BURDOCK will help the body eliminate and strengthen the liver and blood.
ROSEMARY to improve general circulation and raise spirits.

Decoction
WILLOW BARK (an anti-inflammatory) with a pinch of ginger.

Foot bath
GINGER OR MUSTARD to warm the body and improve blood circulation.

RESULTS OF MONITORING

First week: Little improvement but the baths feel good. Add exercise, squeezing a tennis ball and a walk every two days. Sing and dance round house on cold rainy days.
After two months: Slow improvement, whole circulation improved, chilblains gone. Joints need oil; eat oily fish twice a week. Will repeat for another three months.
After three more months: Last month when the weather changed (west wind), had a bout, but it was less severe than previously. Took willow and ginger decoction for over a week. Now it is better again. Raise general expectations of self to avoid depression. Affirmations useful.

CAUTION

If you are at all uncertain of the meaning of symptoms, go to a professional for an accurate diagnosis. If there is a high fever, sudden changes in the condition or it responds unexpectedly to treatment, seek help. Fevers above 102°F (39°C) in infants always need urgent professional attention.

OBSERVATION

Exercise important. Eat more vegetables, eat more often. Vegetable soups easy, quick, and warming. Hand baths wonderful: I have experimented with cedarwood and sandalwood, which are similar to juniper in effect but with different smells. I prefer lavender before bed, to help me sleep soundly. Foot baths a real find, warming the whole body and greatly improving mobility and motivation. After a foot bath, I put on two pairs of socks and can face the outside world. If I get cold, it only takes an eight-minute soak to warm me up again.

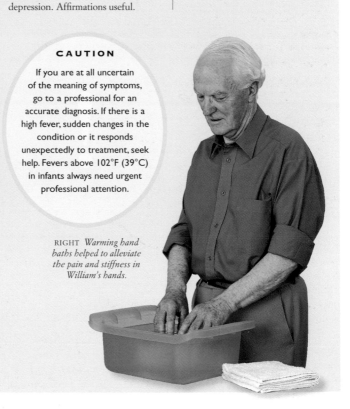

RIGHT *Warming hand baths helped to alleviate the pain and stiffness in William's hands.*

Skin

The skin is the largest organ of the body, eliminating waste matter through sweat and helping maintain normal temperature. It also has to contain and protect the internal organs, yet still be sensitive and subtle enough to feel, touch, and inform. It does all this by continually growing and renewing itself. Many skin conditions are a reflection of internal imbalance, so both internal and external remedies are used. Flower remedies may also prove helpful.

TO KEEP THE SKIN HEALTHY

- Nutrition (especially fresh fruit, root and green vegetable).
- Hygiene.
- Exercise.
- Protection (avoid strong sunshine).
- Water (drink 8 glasses each day).

HERBAL STRATEGIES

Internal medicines
- Alteratives and lymphatic deobstructants.
- Softening remedies.
- Antiallergic and calming remedies.
- Circulatory remedies.

External remedies
- Antiseptic and anti-inflammatory lotions.
- Drawing creams and poultices.
- Cooling lotions.
- Oils and ointments.
- Astringents.

ECZEMA

An itchy rash composed of tiny blisters filled with clear fluid. May be quite dry or weeping. Usually associated with allergies. It may be caused by contact with metals, clothing, detergents, or other substances. Diagnosed from the distribution of the rash.

Applications
- Camomile and marigold creams.
- Bran or oat baths.
- If weeping: lotion or paste of mallow and sage.
- If the skin is cracked, try using comfrey ointment.
- If very dry: marigold infused oil after the bath.

Internal medicines
- Dandelion root and burdock or yellow dock.
- Valerian or camomile for irritability and sleeplessness.

Other measures
- Wear loose, natural fabrics.
- Avoid soap. Use emulsifying or emollient creams to clean the skin.
- Avoid foods with additives, especially colorings.
- Check for allergies.
- Treat any digestive disorders.
- Evening primrose oil performs well in trials. Adult dose: 6 capsules per day.
- Impatiens and crab apple flower remedies are useful.

Consult a professional if the rash becomes infected.

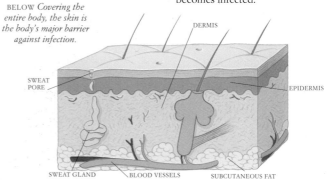

BELOW *Covering the entire body, the skin is the body's major barrier against infection.*

DERMIS

SWEAT PORE

EPIDERMIS

SWEAT GLAND   BLOOD VESSELS   SUBCUTANEOUS FAT

PSORIASIS

Characterized by thick, dry flaky patches, often hereditary, and often triggered by stress. The following herbal remedies will help to keep it under control.

Applications
• Infused oils of nettles, marigold, comfrey, or St. John's wort.
Internal medicines
• 2 parts yellow dock, 2 parts burdock, and 1 part licorice. Persist.
• Add valerian if stress is a factor.
Other measures
• Take fish oils internally.
• Sunshine.
• Dead sea salt baths help.
• Avoid alcohol.
See a professional if joint pain is involved.

ACNE

Large, red spots mostly on the face and back, usually starting during adolescence.

Applications
• Aloe vera, lemon juice, sage.
• Oat and marigold washes, pastes, and poultices.
• Comfrey cream for the scars.
Internal medicines
• Marigold flowers and burdock leaf.
• Add echinacea if sore or badly infected.
• Add agnus castus if hormonally linked.
Other measures
• Eat plenty of fresh fruit and vegetables.

ACNE ROSACEA

Spots associated with very red skin on the face.

Applications
• Aloe vera, rosewater.
Other measures
• Avoid alcohol, sugar, and caffeine.
(*see also Acne left*)

ATHLETE'S FOOT AND FUNGAL INFECTIONS

Causes the skin to become red, flaky, and itchy.

Applications
• Garlic, thyme, aloe vera, and marigold.
Other measures
• Can often be improved by an "anti-candida" diet (*see The Immune System, pp. 124–125*).

WARTS

Lumps on the skin caused by a virus.

Applications
• Fresh garlic, lemon skin juice, sap from dandelion flower stalks.

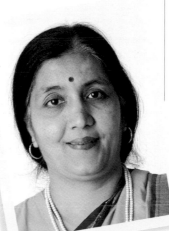

Can be persistent, so try different combinations of remedies.
See a professional for genital warts.

HERPES, COLD SORES, AND SHINGLES

Sore, burning, and itching patches followed by blisters.

Applications
• St. John's wort tincture or infused oil; aloe vera.
• Cayenne cream for post-shingles neuralgia.
Internal medicines
• St. John's wort, long term.
• Echinacea taken during attacks.
See a professional if a fever develops or if shingles appears near the eyes.

HAIR LOSS AND SCALP PROBLEMS

Stress usually causes patchy hair loss, but it is temporary. Male-pattern baldness may improve with herbal remedies.
See a professional if losing body hair.

Applications
• Rosemary, nettle, sage.
Internal medicines
• Rosemary for circulation.
• Horsetail for minerals.
• Valerian or skullcap for stress.
Other measures
• B vitamins.
• Gentle scalp massage.
• Head or shoulder stands.

LEFT *Use both internal and external remedies to keep your skin healthy.*

Bones and Joints

The bones provide a rigid framework for the muscles and serve to protect the internal organs. They are not unchanging, however: bone is continually breaking down and being replaced in the same way as other body tissues. If the body is inactive, the bones will become relatively weak and unable to withstand much stress. Bone density and strength can be increased with only a small amount of exercise, which will reduce the risk of fractures. Similarly, joints can be kept healthy with regular gentle exercise.

LEFT *The skeleton is the body's framework, providing shape and protection.*

HERBAL STRATEGIES

Internal medicines
• Anti-inflammatories.
• Diuretics.
• Healing to promote bone and nerve healing.

External remedies
• Warming liniments.
• Cooling compresses.
• Healing, promoting bone healing.

SPRAINS

Sprains occur when the ligaments surrounding a joint are torn as a result of excessive demands being made on the joint.

Applications
• Comfrey and cabbage.
Other measures
• Rest.
• Cold packs or compress straight-way to reduce swelling.
• Try alternating hot and cold packs if the pain persists for more than a few days.

• For old injuries massage with liniments of comfrey and warming herbs such as cayenne and ginger.

OSTEOPOROSIS

Brittle bones. A common cause of broken bones in elderly people. More common in post-menopausal women. Sometimes hereditary.

Internal medicines
• Parsley, horsetail, comfrey, and nettles to improve the utilization of calcium .
• Parsley, fennel, agnus castus and sage help hormone levels.
Other measures
• Research shows that exercise is the best way of strengthening bones. Do something daily.
• Avoid excess alcohol and coffee. Stop smoking.
• Reduce animal protein, including meat and milk products. Soy products contain vegetable protein and more calcium than milk. Dark green vegetables are excellent.

TO KEEP BONES AND JOINTS HEALTHY

• Nutrition (especially oily fish and green vegetables).
• Gentle exercise (with weights).
• Good posture.
• Moderate exposure to sunshine (vitamin D).
• Good circulation.

RHEUMATOID ARTHRITIS AND INFLAMMATORY JOINT PAIN

Hot, swollen joints. Usually widespread and affecting small joints such as the fingers.

Applications
• Aloe vera, cabbage leaves, comfrey.
Internal medicines
• Willow bark, celery seed, meadowsweet, marigold, Siberian ginseng.
Other measures
• Alternating hot and cold packs.
• Baths with Epsom salt and rosemary or thyme essential oils.
• Vitamin C and fish oils.
• Dietary restrictions. These vary according to the individual; monitor your symptoms.
• Keep mind and body active and flexible. Try crossword puzzles, yoga, and gentle exercise.
See a professional for persistent, inflammatory joint pain. Early treatment will prevent permanent joint damage.

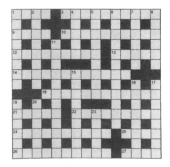

BELOW *If you suffer from joint pain, try to keep your mind active with brain stretching activities.*

OSTEOARTHRITIS AND STIFF JOINTS

Stiff painful joints, worse after immobility and in cold weather.

Applications
• Warming herbs such as ginger, cayenne, and thyme.
Internal medicines
• As for rheumatoid arthritis, adding circulatory remedies.
Other measures
• Physiotherapy, massage, salt baths.
• Hot and cold packs.
• Mineral supplements.
• Drink 2 tsp (10ml) cider vinegar and one of honey in hot water daily.
• Exercise that avoids putting weight on the joint, for example swimming.

GOUT

Painful, hot, swollen joints, usually the big toe or thumb.

Applications
• Cabbage leaf, cider vinegar.
Internal medicines
• *(see rheumatoid arthritis)*; nettle tea.
Other measures
• Low-protein diet. Avoid alcohol, red meat, kidney, liver, and seafood.
• A vegetarian diet will help gout.

BACK PAIN

Back pain can be very difficult to treat successfully without specialist help, but the following measures will usually improve the condition.

Applications
• Massage with St. John's wort infused oil.
• Cayenne plasters.

Internal medicines
• Willow bark and celery seed.
• Valerian or cramp bark to reduce spasm.
Other measures
• Exercise is always beneficial for chronic pain, but see a physiotherapist, yoga teacher, chiropractor, or osteopath for specific exercises, which will improve the condition without adding more strain to the back.
• Check posture, seating positions, height and angle of work surfaces.

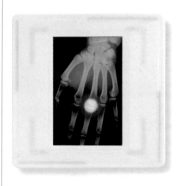

ABOVE *Alleviate joint pain with alternating hot and cold packs.*

BROKEN BONES

Broken bones should, of course, be properly set, after an X-ray to confirm the diagnosis.

Other measures
• Comfrey internally and externally will speed bone healing.
• Marigold and plantain will promote healing in general.
• Massage above and below the plaster to maintain a good circulation. Twiddle toes or fingers to keep some strength and mobility.

Circulatory System

The circulatory system comprises the heart, blood, and blood vessels, which create a continuous flow of blood around the body. The heart pumps the blood, which carries nutrients and oxygen, through the arteries to the organs and tissues, from where the veins and muscles carry it back to the heart and then to the lungs to be reoxygenated. Many organs play a part in this cycle, including the kidneys, which filter and maintain water balance, the liver and bone marrow, which make red blood cells, and the spleen, which provides lymphocytes.

TO KEEP CIRCULATION HEALTHY

- Good diet. Warming foods are especially useful.
- Gentle skin brushing all over the body for overall circulation.
- Healthy kidney function.

- Regular exercise that produces a light sweat.
- Open-hearted, or whole-hearted activity. Singing and kite flying.
- Avoid excess stresses and smoking.

In medieval times the heart was assigned to the Sun and pictured radiating out warmth, nourishment, and emotional good will to the rest of the body.

HERBAL STRATEGIES

- Strengthen the heart.
- Strengthen blood vessels.
- Warming.
- Nourish the blood.
- Clear the blood and blood vessels.
- Relaxing nervines.

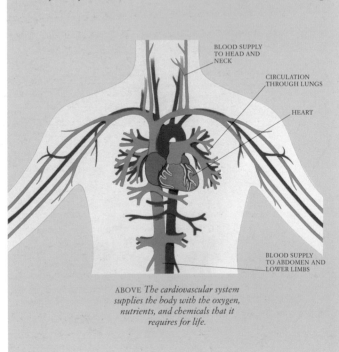

BLOOD SUPPLY TO HEAD AND NECK

CIRCULATION THROUGH LUNGS

HEART

BLOOD SUPPLY TO ABDOMEN AND LOWER LIMBS

ABOVE *The cardiovascular system supplies the body with the oxygen, nutrients, and chemicals that it requires for life.*

POOR CIRCULATION

Cold hands and feet, white finger, tendency to chilblains.

Internal medicines
- Rosemary, cayenne, cinnamon, angelica, hawthorn. Ginger for sudden chills.

Applications
- Warming herbs as above.

Other measures
- Regular exercise, cold showers.
- Stop smoking.

VARICOSE VEINS

Aches, swelling, and inflammation respond to treatment.

Internal medicines
• Yarrow with hawthorn and other circulatory medicines. Dandelion root.
Applications
• Comfrey, yarrow, witch hazel. Marigold for inflammations.
Other measures
• Raise the foot of the bed.
• Regular toe twiddling and bicycling on your back. Yoga.
• Support stockings.
• Vitamin E

HIGH CHOLESTEROL, HYPERLIPIDEMIA

Revealed by blood test. Contributes to heart disease.

Internal medicines
• Garlic, oats, hawthorn, linden flowers, gingko, dandelion root are all useful additions to the diet, or taken as a remedy. See each herb for specific methods and uses.
Other measures
• Diet: cut down on animal fats (fatty meats, eggs, milk products), alcohol, sugar, and hydrogenated vegetable fats.
• Virgin olive oil, oily fish, globe artichokes, apples, and purslane are beneficial.
• Regular exercise.

ANEMIA

Lack of iron, pallor, tiredness. Due to blood loss or poor iron absorption. Common in pregnancy and when breast-feeding. May follow a viral infection.

Internal medicines
• Nettles, parsley, Chinese angelica, dandelion root, dock, and burdock can all be added to the diet or taken as teas, tonic wine, syrup decoctions, or tincture.
Other measures
• Vitamin C.
• Seaweeds, red meat, watercress, and apricots are beneficial. Reduce coffee consumption.

YARROW

See a professional if anemia persists.

HIGH BLOOD PRESSURE

High blood pressure can increase the risk of heart attacks and strokes.

Internal medicines
• Add hawthorn, yarrow, and garlic to the diet or as internal remedies.
• Nettles or dandelion leaf as diuretics.
• Try valerian root and flower remedies if stress induced.
Other measures
• Reduce salt and alcohol.
• Stop smoking.
• Reduce excess weight.
See also High Cholesterol (above) and Stress (p.127)
Moderately high blood pressure can be treated with these measures. Do not stop medication without first seeking professional guidance.

GARLIC CLOVE

LOW BLOOD PRESSURE

This condition may be due to anemia or exhaustion. Can cause dizziness, fainting, tinnitus, and a constant wish to lie down. It is always worth checking for an underlying cause in these cases. Constitutional low blood pressure without symptoms does not need treating.

Internal medicines
• Cayenne, rosemary, ginseng.
Other measures
• Very low-salt diets can precipitate low blood pressure.
• Add seaweeds to the diet.

STROKE

Damage to the circulation in the brain causing paralysis on one side of the body. May be due to weakening blood vessels or blood clots. Attacks may be sudden, or develop slowly over a few hours. Transient strokes with symptoms such as fainting and subsequent weakness in one part of the body are a warning sign, and should be checked by a professional.

Internal medicines
• Yarrow and gingko will reduce the risk of another attack.
• Take herbs for high blood pressure, as it is a contributory cause of low blood pressure.
• Siberian ginseng will assist regeneration.
Applications
• Massage with gentle warming (not hot) herbs such as rosemary, angelica, fennel, and juniper.
Other measures
• Diet as for high blood pressure and high cholesterol.
• Gentle exercise and passive movement of paralyzed limbs.
• Provide plenty of stimulation, in order to maintain the effort toward recovery and an enthusiasm for life.

115

Urinary System

The urinary system consists of the kidneys, in which the blood is filtered of waste products and urine is formed, the ureters, which transport the urine from the kidneys, the bladder, which stores the urine, and the urethra, through which urine is excreted. To maintain a healthy system, we need to drink plenty of water. Elimination is a key factor in many conditions including skin problems, arthritis, and gout. Soothing kidney herbs such as cornsilk and marshmallow are nearly always applicable and are put into many remedies.

TO KEEP THE URINARY SYSTEM HEALTHY

- Nutrition (especially green vegetables).
- Water (drink 8 glasses each day).
- Exercise (walking and bending).
- Pelvic and lower back exercise.
- Stress management.

HERBAL STRATEGIES

- Diuretics.
- Urinary antiseptics.
- Demulcents.
- Anti-inflammatories.
- Hormone balancing (prostate).

Urine should be slightly acid as it eliminates the acid produced by the body's metabolic functions. Take cranberry to alkalize it, a teaspoon of vinegar in water to make it more acid. Always answer a need to urinate as soon as possible – as ignoring it can cause problems later on in life.

DIURETICS

Diuretics are substances that increase the amount of urine produced by the kidneys, thus helping to remove excess fluid from the body.

They are used to:
- Flush out the bladder and kidneys.
- Flush wastes from the body, especially in arthritis and skin disease.
- Relieve edema and water retention, with other herbs to address the cause.
- Treat high blood pressure.

Herbal diuretics include dandelion leaf and root, burdock root, elderflower, fennel, parsley, nettle, and cleavers.

CYSTITIS

Inflammation of the bladder lining, causing a burning pain on urination, with urgency and frequency. Can be related to diet, sexual activity, spermicidal creams, and bubble baths, or to an infection. It is more common in women than men since it is easier for bacteria to spread from the rectum to the urethra.

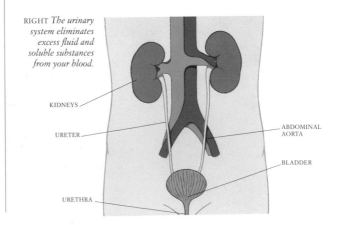

RIGHT *The urinary system eliminates excess fluid and soluble substances from your blood.*

KIDNEYS

URETER

ABDOMINAL AORTA

BLADDER

URETHRA

Internal medicines
• Diuretics, especially dandelion leaf.
• Urinary antiseptics: celery seed, fennel, angelica, thyme.
• Demulcent, soothing remedies, especially marshmallow.
• Make a tea using one herb from each category, and drink several cups a day.

Other measures
• Drink plenty of water.
• Cranberry juice, bilberry juice, and lemon barley water are helpful.
• Take 1 tsp (5ml) of bicarbonate of soda (baking soda) dissolved in a glass of warm water every 6 hours.
• Good toilet hygiene: always wipe from front to back to avoid bacteria spreading from the anus to the bladder.
• Empty bladder and wash immediately after sexual intercourse, but don't use soap as this may promote irritation.
• Avoid wearing synthetic underwear and pantyhose.
• Avoid sugar, very spicy foods, coffee, tea, and cola drinks.
• Diet should include lots of vegetables and minimal meat.
See a professional if there is blood in your urine or if you develop mid-back pain and fever, indicating that the infection has spread up the ureters toward the kidneys.

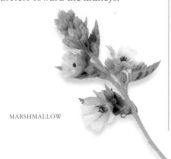
MARSHMALLOW

CHRONIC CYSTITIS AND IRRITABLE BLADDER
Recurrent bladder pain with low back pain, urinary frequency, and painful urination suggests a chronic inflammation of the bladder or urinary tract. Seek professional advice immediately.

Internal medicines
• Marigold, St. John's wort, yarrow, and horsetail.
• (*See Cystitis, above.*)

Other measures
• Alternating hot and cold packs.

KIDNEY STONES AND GRAVEL
Pain and tenderness in the mid back that moves down and round to the bladder as stones are passed. This pain can be severe. Gravel or small stones in the urine. May be hereditary. May be caused by excessive intake of calcium in antacid preparations.

Internal medicines
• Marshmallow leaf with diuretics such as parsley and dandelion leaf.
• Cornsilk.

Other measures
• A ginger compress can be used to ease the pain.
• Drink plenty of low-calcium bottled water.
Different types of stones require different regimes. Check with a professional if in doubt.

ENLARGED PROSTATE
Difficult urination, loss of force, dribbling, and increased frequency of urination. The swollen prostate blocks the passage of urine from the bladder. May lead to cystitis. Common in older men.

Internal medicines
• Nettle root, willow bark, saw palmetto, Siberian ginseng.

Other measures
• Pumpkin seeds, 4 tsp (20ml) daily, may be eaten with muesli.
• Flower pollen.
• Soy products, evening primrose oil, and oily fish helpful.
Prostate symptoms should be checked by a professional. A simple blood test will exclude prostate cancer.

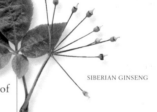
SIBERIAN GINSENG

INCONTINENCE
Loss of control in the bladder often as a result of an urinary tract disorder. Common in the elderly as the sphincter muscles lose tone.

Internal medicines
• Horsetail, yarrow, agrimony, St. John's wort.

Other measures
• Exercising the bladder sphincter muscles – tightening and relaxing.
• Stop smoking
If these measures don't help, seek further investigations.

Respiratory System

The lungs take in air with each breath, absorbing the nutrient gases we need and exhaling the gases we do not need. Breathing should be a smooth automatic, effortless process, with slight movement from the inside of the collar bone at the top of the lungs (not the shoulders) to the abdomen, which moves with the action of the diaphragm. Breathing oxygenates the blood and brain, giving us the energy that we need.

TO KEEP THE RESPIRATORY SYSTEM HEALTHY

- Nutrition.
- Unpolluted, moist air (humidify air conditioning).
- Exercise (brisk walking or swimming).
- Singing.
- Breathing exercises.
- Protection (wear a mask in poor air conditions).

HERBAL STRATEGIES

- Anti-catarrhals.
- Mucous membrane restoratives.
- Expectorants – soothing, stimulating, or antibacterial.
- Lung restoratives.
- Antiallergic remedies.
- Inhalants and chest rubs.

Defenses of the respiratory system include: the hairs in the nose that warm and filter air; sneezing that removes irritants; contraction of the bronchi that limits inhalation of irritants; production of mucus that coats and helps to cough up irritants or infection. Herbal remedies work in conjunction with these defenses to help restore healthy functioning of the respiratory system.

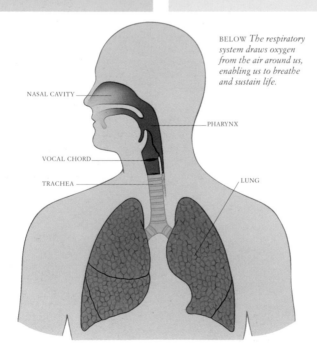

NASAL CAVITY

PHARYNX

VOCAL CHORD

TRACHEA

LUNG

BELOW *The respiratory system draws oxygen from the air around us, enabling us to breathe and sustain life.*

COLDS AND FLU

Try to respond to the very first signs of colds and flu (sneezing, watery eyes, sore throat, runny nose).
Internal medicines and inhalants.
- Elderflower, yarrow, peppermint, garlic, sage, ginger, cinnamon.
- Echinacea if infected, or if a fever develops.
Other measures
- Take vitamin C, around 2 or 3 grams, daily.

CHRONIC CATARRH

Blocked or discharging nose, post-nasal drip, sinus pain, and headaches around and above the eyes. May lead to middle-ear congestion and earache.

Applications
- Cayenne cream over the sinuses.
- For earache use drops of garlic or St. John's wort infused oil.

Internal medicines and inhalants
- As for colds. Camomile, rosemary, or thyme inhalants.

Other measures
- Vitamin C.
- Try cutting out milk products or wheat.
- Nasal douche with saltwater.
- Keep the head warm in cold weather.

HAY FEVER

Allergic reaction to airborne allergen (e.g., grass pollen) that occurs in the eyes, nose, and throat.

Internal medicines and inhalants
- Elderflower, eyebright, garlic, yarrow, camomile, nettles, sage.
- For sneezing; elderflower or eyebright in saltwater as nose drops.
- Eye baths – camomile, elderflower, eyebright.

Other measures
- Inhale from a bottle of camomile essential oil for quick relief.
- Local honey, 3 tsp (15ml) daily.
- Diet: cut out milk products during the season; eat plenty of fresh vegetables.

COUGHS AND BRONCHITIS

Most coughs require a mixture of remedies. Vary the proportions according to need.

Applications
- Chest rubs based on infused oils of garlic or thyme.

Internal medicines for productive coughs (with sticky phlegm)
- Thyme, coltsfoot, mullein, garlic, elecampane, angelica, sage.

- For infected coughs (with green phlegm), add garlic or thyme.

Internal medicines for dry, irritable coughs
- Marshmallow, comfrey, licorice, coltsfoot, honey, and syrups.

ELECAMPANE

- Add valerian or camomile for nervous coughs.

Internal medicine for persistent coughs and chronic bronchitis
- Coltsfoot, mullein, elecampane, sage taken long term.

Other measures
- Cut out milk products.
- Stop smoking.

Herbal tobaccos may be helpful (see *Coltsfoot, pp. 96–97*).

See a professional for a persistent dry, unproductive cough with no obvious cause, and for bronchitis in small children, as it can quickly progress to pneumonia.

EMPHYSEMA

Damaged lungs exacerbated by cigarette smoking. Symptoms are severe breathlessness and fast breathing, barrel-shaped chest, and often a persistent, chronic cough.

- Take regular garlic to keep lung infections at bay.
- Herbs for persistent cough are helpful.
- A gentle postural drainage may be useful if it does not overtax the strength of the patient.
- Warming oils rubbed around the base of the ribs and covered with a large crepe bandage alleviate the symptoms of some sufferers.

ASTHMA

Recurrent attacks of breathlessness, wheezing, and tension in the lungs, often following coughs, exercise, or stress. Often caused by allergies (*see p. 124*). Most attacks pass naturally, but a severe attack can be dangerous and will need immediate professional help.

Applications
- As for coughs (*see above*). Massage into the back with a gentle circular motion.

Internal medicines
- Thyme, elecampane, mullein, garlic.
- Valerian or skullcap for nervous asthma.
- Camomile for allergic asthma.
- Cinnamon and dandelion leaf are often helpful additions.

Other measures
- Avoid or remove allergens and other triggers.
- Keep the air damp by using sprays and vaporizers with a few drops of lavender, thyme, or eucalyptus essential oils.
- To prevent dehydration, drink plenty of water .
- Breathing exercises to strengthen the lungs, singing, swimming, blowing up balloons.
- A low-salt diet excluding artificial coloring, monosodium glutamate, and cheap wines.
- Exclude all milk products, especially if sinus troubles or eczema are also present.

Reproductive System

The reproductive system develops during puberty. The changes of adolescence, the menstrual cycle, and, later, of menopause and declining fertility are stressful times, both physically and emotionally, and can benefit from certain herbal remedies. Stress has a profound effect on the balance of the sex hormones, and emotional health can be improved with herbs and this in turn can increase fertility. There are many herbal remedies particularly associated with the sex organs.

TO KEEP THE REPRODUCTIVE SYSTEM HEALTHY

• Nutrition (especially nuts, seeds, wholegrains, and green vegetables).
• Avoid excessive stress.
• Pelvic exercise (dancing and belly dancing).
• Maintain correct weight for height.

B-COMPLEX
TABLETS

HERBAL STRATEGIES

• Relax tension in the womb.
• Clear water retention.
• Rebalance the hormones.
• Strengthen and tone the organs of reproduction.
• Rebalance the relationship between nervous system and hormonal system.

BELOW *The male and female reproductive system produce sperm and egg cells, necessary for the creation of new life.*

PREMENSTRUAL SYNDROME

Irritability, depression, water retention, bloating, and painful breasts for a week or so before menstruation occurs.

Internal medicines
• Agnus castus.
• Add camomile, linden flowers, or skullcap for nervousness.
• Add sage, fennel, or marshmallow for breast pain.
• Parsley or dandelion leaf for water retention and swollen breasts.

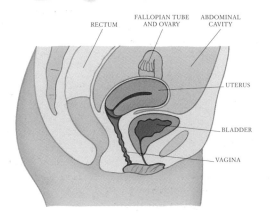

RECTUM
FALLOPIAN TUBE AND OVARY
ABDOMINAL CAVITY
UTERUS
BLADDER
VAGINA

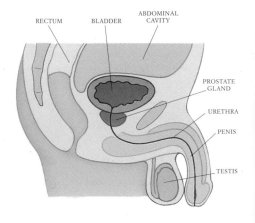

RECTUM
BLADDER
ABDOMINAL CAVITY
PROSTATE GLAND
URETHRA
PENIS
TESTIS

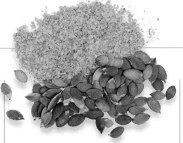

WHOLE WHEAT BREAD
AND PUMPKIN SEEDS

Other measures
• For low blood sugar, eat little and often and avoid coffee.
• Evening primrose oil can help the physical symptoms.
• Many women find vitamin B_6 helpful. It may be better to take B complex tablets.

PERIOD PAIN

Periods pains are often characterized by a dull ache or cramping pains in the lower part of the abdomen.

Applications
• Ginger compress or hot water bottle to the lower abdomen.
• Hot foot bath.
Internal medicines
• Marigold, raspberry leaves, motherwort, St. John's wort, cramp bark, peppermint, yarrow, Chinese angelica.
• A little ginger added to the above teas is always beneficial.
Take these medicines for two weeks before your period.
• Severe pain can often be controlled by freely taking cramp bark with a little ginger.

HEAVY PERIODS

These may be due to iron deficiency, fibroids, an intra-uterine device (I.U.D.), or hormonal imbalance.

Internal medicines
• Raspberry leaf, lady's mantle, shepherd's purse.
• Add nettles for anemia.
See a professional for bleeding between periods.

MENOPAUSAL PROBLEMS

Hot sweats, depression, mood swings, and other symptoms associated with more irregular and infrequent periods. There is usually no need to take Hormone Replacement Therapy (H.R.T.).

Internal medicines
• Agnus castus, sage, parsley, motherwort, St. John's wort, licorice, Chinese angelica.
• Cold sage tea is effective for most cases of hot flushes.

VAGINAL THRUSH

A white discharge with itching is usually due to thrush (*Candida albicans*). It should not be ignored.

Applications
Washes, ointments, creams, and douches.
• Aloe vera, marigold, raspberry leaves, garlic.
• Hormonal remedies may prove to be helpful.
• Live yogurt is helpful and soothing.
Other measures
• Avoid pantyhose.
• For persistent cases follow an anti-candida diet (*see p. 125*).

LOSS OF SEX DRIVE AND IMPOTENCE

This happens to everyone at some time or other. It may be due to prolonged stress and anxiety, tiredness, or to hormonal imbalance and some drugs.

Internal medicines
• Siberian ginseng. Burdock root for elderly people.
• Agnus castus for women.
• Circulatory remedies may help men unable to achieve an erection: hawthorn, cayenne, ginger.
• Mint, basil, ginger, mace, and cinnamon may all help short-term. A pleasant liqueur can be made by soaking 1 tbsp (15ml) of each in 2½ cups (600ml) of brandy. Take 3–4 tsp (15–20ml) when needed.

INFERTILITY

May be due to blocked fallopian tubes, hormonal imbalances, or a low sperm count. Often no specific cause can be found. The following herbs are often helpful:

Internal medicines
• For women: sage, lady's mantle, and marigold. Marigold often helps in cases of blockage. Agnus castus for hormonal imbalance.
• For men: Siberian ginseng and sarsaparilla.
• Cayenne if circulation is poor, or for pelvic congestion.
Other measures
• General health measures; good diet and exercise.
• Diet should be low in animal fats and high in fresh vegetables.
• Zinc is the best nutritional supplement. Pumpkin seeds, aduki beans, pine nuts, and wheatgerm are excellent sources of zinc. Oats are also beneficial.
• Smoking and alcohol can both reduce fertility.

Digestive System

The same epithelial cells (with variations) coat the whole digestive system, from the mouth to the stomach, intestines, and colon. The process of digestion starts when food is chewed, and salivary enzymes are released. It continues as digestive juices in the stomach break down the food still further, and ends after the substances that the body needs have been absorbed and the waste products are excreted via the anus as feces. It takes at least 24 hours for this process to be completed. Poor appetite is normal during some illnesses when the body spends energy on healing rather than digesting.

TO KEEP THE DIGESTIVE SYSTEM HEALTHY

• Nutrition (varied diet with plenty of fiber).
• Regular bowel movement.
• Reduce tension (emotion upsets the stomach).

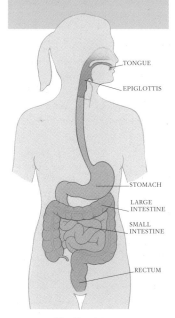

ABOVE *The digestive system ingests food and eliminates solid waste from the body.*

TONGUE
EPIGLOTTIS
STOMACH
LARGE INTESTINE
SMALL INTESTINE
RECTUM

HERBAL STRATEGIES

• Demulcents.
• Aromatic carminatives.
• Bitters.
• Anti-inflammatories.
• Antispasmodics.
• Astringents.
• Laxatives.

Defenses of the system are reflex coughing (if something is stuck in the throat), vomiting, and rapid evacuation.

SORE MOUTH AND THROAT, GUM DISEASE

Includes soreness inside the mouth and on or around the tongue. Gums may be inflamed.
• Sage is the most useful remedy – in toothpaste and as a mouthwash and gargle. A pinch of salt will help.
• When making a gargle, add marshmallow (tea, decoction, or tincture) for extreme soreness and mouth ulcers.
• Add echinacea (tea, decoction, or tincture) or a couple of cloves for toothache and abscess.

• Add marigold (tea, decoction, or tincture) for tonsillitis and thrush.
• Add a pinch of cayenne for laryngitis and sore throats that are worse in the cold.

ACID STOMACH

Burning pain in the stomach after eating, heartburn, acid reflux, poor appetite. May lead to ulcers. The inside of the stomach should have a mucous coating to protect it from the acids of digestion. Demulcent remedies will help restore it.

Internal medicines
• Meadowsweet with comfrey and camomile.
• Peppermint, fennel, cinnamon.
• Demulcent remedies before meals: marshmallow, slippery elm, licorice, carrot juice, cabbage water or juice.
• Add echinacea if the symptoms are severe and persistent, or thyme as an antiseptic.
Other measures
• Stop smoking, reduce alcohol.
• Avoid spicy and fatty foods.
• Eat slowly.
• Papaya extract is helpful.

NAUSEA

Feelings of sickness in the upper abdomen, throat, or chest. May be followed by vomiting.

• Ginger in all forms, tea, tincture, decoction, candied, or just chewing a small piece of fresh root helps to alleviate nausea. A ginger compress over the stomach helps if the nausea is due to tension and spasm.

• For persistent nausea, use liver remedies and seek advice.

LIVER DISORDERS

Modern life is hard on the liver. Excess alcohol, rich and processed foods, pollution, and many medicines all put extra stress on the liver, as do suppressed anger and resentment. Symptoms include indigestion, intolerance of fats, low alcohol tolerance, feelings of heaviness and nausea, constipation, pale stools, itchy skin, depression, unreasonable anger, and jaundice. Liver remedies should be included in regimes for allergies, arthritis, and skin problems.

Internal medicines

• Dandelion root and burdock are the most important remedies.

• Add yellow dock, angelica, rosemary, sage, or thyme according to the specific symptoms.

Other measures

• Diet should be light and include plenty of fresh fruit and vegetables.

• Globe artichokes, garlic, and olive oil are helpful.

• Bending and stretching exercises.

• Let out anger safely by doing something creative.

See a professional if symptoms persist or worsen.

GALLSTONES

Gallstones are stones that form in the gallbladder.

Internal medicines

• As for liver disorders with an emphasis on rosemary or yellow dock.

Other measures

• Fresh apple juice, oats, and leafy vegetables. The stones can be flushed out but this is best carried out under the guidance of a professional.

IRRITABLE BOWEL

ROSEMARY

Indigestion and abdominal pain, bloating, and wind. Morning diarrhea. Constipation alternates with diarrhea. Mucus in the stools. Irritable bowel is becoming more common, caused by stress, food intolerance, and gut infections. It commonly starts after a course of strong antibiotics.

Internal medicines

• For stress and pain: valerian or camomile.

• For flatulence and bloating: peppermint, sage, elecampane, and fennel are good.

• For diarrhea that is persistent, add raspberry leaves or meadowsweet.

BURDOCK

• For persistent constipation try adding dock.

• Always add a demulcent: comfrey, marshmallow, or slippery elm.

Other measures

• Eat foods rich in soluble fiber: steamed leafy vegetables and oats. Be careful with "added bran" cereals as they may be too heavy. See a professional if there is blood in the stools or a sudden onset of symptoms with no previous history of indigestion.

DIARRHEA

For chronic diarrhea refer to Irritable Bowel (*see above*). For acute diarrhea arising from food poisoning or infection, take:

• Yellow dock with cinnamon or ginger.

Other measures

Drink plenty of liquid to prevent dehydration. A pint of boiled water containing a pinch of salt and 2 tsp (10ml) of honey makes a good emergency fluid. Drink freely.

CONSTIPATION

Constipation is most often caused by eating a diet that is low in fiber or by not drinking enough fluids.

• Dandelion root, yellow dock, aloe vera leaf.

• Add valerian or camomile for colicky pain and stress constipation.

Other measures

• Eat high-fiber foods; whole-grain bread, oats, and leafy vegetables.

• Take regular exercise.

Immune System

The means by which the body is able to protect itself from harmful organisms and maintain a balanced chemistry is known as the immune system. It includes the lymphatic system, which carries nutrients, drains waste products, and produces lymphocytes and antibodies to combat disease. Swollen "glands" at the neck, groin, and armpit during disease are signs that the lymph nodes are working to capacity. A weakened immune system is indicated by small but persistent minor infections, sudden allergy, or food intolerance, and general tiredness. Some illness may be regarded as misguided attempts by the body to protect itself.

TO KEEP THE IMMUNE SYSTEM HEALTHY

- Nutrition.
- Plenty of fluids.
- Exercise.
- Avoid excessive internal and external stress.
- Emotional balance.
- Regular elimination via skin, kidney, and bowel.

HERBAL STRATEGIES

- Immune restoratives and stimulants.
- Lymphatic deobstructants.
- Relaxing nervines and antidepressants.
- Assisting remedies.
- Fever remedies.
- Antiseptics, antivirals, and antibiotics.
- Anti-inflammatories.

ALLERGIES

A hypersensitivity to specific materials, foods, or other substances including nuts, fish, eggs, seafood, pollens, dust mites, some plants, insect bites, and stings, nickel, sulfur (used to preserve foods), penicillin, aspirin, food colorings and preservatives, chemicals, and tampons. Reactions only arise on second or subsequent exposure to the allergen.

PERSISTENT MINOR INFECTIONS

Caused by weak immune system.

Internal medicines

- Garlic, echinacea, Siberian ginseng, sage.
- Add marigold to help relieve chronic tonsillitis and swollen lymph nodes.
- Use fever herbs; elderflowers, yarrow, marigold, and thyme to deal with the symptoms of fevers and flu. Try to avoid the excessive use of antibiotics. (*See also Sore Throats, p.122.*)

POST-VIRAL EXHAUSTION

Chronic fatigue, depression, and night sweats following a viral infection such as influenza.

- Sage, marigold, echinacea, Siberian ginseng, elecampane, nettles, angelica.
- Cold sage tea for night sweats.
- Cinnamon and angelica for persistent coldness.
- Valerian, skullcap, camomile to promote refreshing sleep.

See a professional if the condition persists for more than a few weeks.

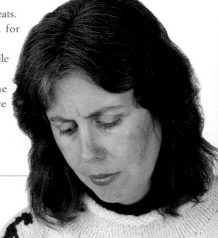

BELOW Take an uplifting herb after a viral infection to raise low spirits.

Symptoms include swelling and inflammation in the mouth, throat, or skin, nettle rash (hives), severe diarrhea and vomiting, asthma, hay fever, eczema, and migraine. A severe reaction can be life-threatening and may need urgent hospital treatment.

Applications
• Camomile, yarrow, plantain, marshmallow.
Internal medicines
• Garlic, nettles, camomile, eyebright.
Other measures
• Coffee has an anti-allergic action. An old treatment for asthma was coffee foot baths. It may be used to help some symptoms, but long-term use is counterproductive.
• Professional herbalists have more powerful herbs at their disposal. Desensitization to an allergen is sometimes possible.
• (*See also Asthma, p.119, Eczema, p.110, and Food Intolerance, p.125.*)

FOOD INTOLERANCE

An inability to digest certain foods properly. May be inherited or acquired. Food intolerance appears to be getting more common, as the body tries to differentiate between food, additive, and pollutants. General symptoms may include indigestion, wind, bloating, heaviness, constipation, or diarrhea. More particular symptoms may be joint pain, eczema, nettle rash, excess catarrh, asthma, low energy, or headaches.

Internal medicines
• Camomile, raspberry leaf, marigold, agrimony, garlic.

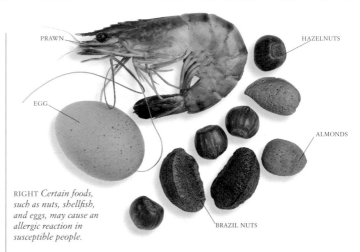

RIGHT Certain foods, such as nuts, shellfish, and eggs, may cause an allergic reaction in susceptible people.

PRAWN

EGG

HAZELNUTS

ALMONDS

BRAZIL NUTS

• Liver remedies: dandelion root, burdock.
Other measures
• Identify suspect foods by keeping a record of your diet and symptoms.
• Intolerance may be masked. The body may seem to be coping but it is only doing so by making a tremendous effort. Suspect any food that you eat in large amounts.
• Cut out the suspect food completely for a month. Then challenge yourself by reintroducing it. Note any change in symptoms.
• If you suspect many foods, or are uncertain of where to start, consult a professional herbalist or nutritionist.

CANDIDIASIS

Candida is a yeast that exists in all digestive systems. Candidiasis is an overgrowth of this yeast, producing wind, bloating, and low energy. It is a sign of a diminished immune system, and

RIGHT Live yogurt has antifungal properties and can be used to treat fungal infections.

may also show as persistent vaginal thrush or fungal infections on the skin, hormone imbalances, and food intolerance. The original imbalance may also be a result of repeated courses of antibiotics.

Internal medicines
• Aloe vera gel, marigold, garlic, raspberry leaf, echinacea.
Other measures
The "anti-candida diet."
• Cut out sugar and all sweet foods, even honey and dried fruit.
• Cut out all yeasty foods: wine, beer, yeast extracts (check labels on prepared foods and vegetarian stocks), matured cheese, and bread (except soda bread).
• Take live yogurt or acidophilus tablets daily.
Continue the treatment for three months. These measures are sufficient for mild cases of candidiasis but for very debilitating cases, or if many food intolerances are suspected, it is best to see a nutritionist or professional herbalist.

The Nervous System

The function of the nervous system is to gather information from outside and within the body and respond in a way that insures survival and results in positive rather than negative experiences. Both types of experience can be stressful, but some stress is necessary to motivate us, test us, and enable us to adapt to new situations. It is the unremitting exposure to stress that can lead to emotional and physical problems. When feeling overstretched, oversensitive, anxious, low-spirited, or overwhelmed, take time to talk to others, listen to your internal needs, and learn relaxation techniques.

TO KEEP THE NERVOUS SYSTEM HEALTHY

• Nutrition (especially vitamin B, found in wholegrains).
• Adequate and restful sleep.
• Emotional balance.

HERBAL STRATEGIES

Defenses include: fight or flight, activity, relaxation techniques, shutting down, and going to sleep.

• Nerve restoratives.
• Relaxing herbs.
• Antidepressants.

HEADACHES

Can be from a number of causes. Sinus headaches are around the eyes and associated with blocked nose or colds. Tension headaches usually feel like a tight band around the forehead and often start with neck tension. Migraines are one-sided and often start with nausea and seeing halos around objects. Other causes to consider are eyestrain, liver problems, allergies, drugs, toxins, air conditioning, and pollution.

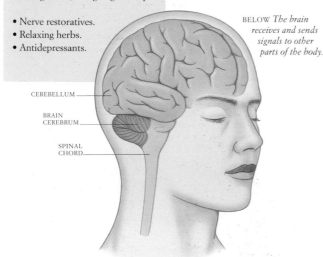

BELOW *The brain receives and sends signals to other parts of the body.*

CEREBELLUM

BRAIN CEREBRUM

SPINAL CHORD

Applications

• For hot-feeling headaches – camomile or lavender compress to forehead and back of the neck.
See a professional if your headaches get worse, include a fever, vomiting, or scalp tenderness, or follow a blow to the head.

Internal medicines
• Camomile, rosemary, skullcap.
• For migraine: rosemary, skullcap, camomile, feverfew. Attacks can sometimes be aborted by holding a little cayenne in the mouth.
• Valerian for any headache arising from anxiety.

NEURALGIA

Burning or sharp pain in the face with tender skin over the area. May result from toothache or exposure to cold drafts.

Applications

• Rosemary or lavender essential oil.
• Cayenne cream if pain is triggered by cold.

Internal medicines
• St. John's wort, skullcap, valerian, rosemary, camomile.

ANXIETY AND STRESS

Inability to relax, thoughts running round, worrying over trivial issues, crying for no reason, irritability, insomnia. Can lead to depression and immune deficiency if not treated seriously.

Internal medicines
• Valerian, camomile, skullcap, lemon balm, sage.

Other measures
• Counseling.
• Reduce caffeine intake – coffee, strong tea, cola drinks.
• Baths with relaxing essential oils: lavender, camomile.
• Regular exercise (to burn off adrenaline).
• Take time off to do nothing in particular – admire the countryside, watch the sea, play with your children. You do have the time, since relaxing will diminish the anxiety and result in a better-organized lifestyle.
• Yoga, meditation, tai chi, or any other relaxation techniques.
• Vitamin B complex.

PANIC ATTACKS

Severe anxiety, palpitations, heart racing, stomach in a knot, dry mouth, sweating, breathing fast and shallow. May be for no obvious reason.
• Regular intake of valerian or camomile.
• Add hawthorn or motherwort for heart racing.
• Valerian and hawthorn drops, to carry with you.

Other measures
• Carry a small bottle of a relaxing

essential oil: lavender, camomile, or neroli. Inhale when feeling panicky.
• Slow your breathing. Breathe calmly into a paper bag if you are hyperventilating.
• Flower remedies: Star of Bethlehem, Bach flower "Rescue Remedy," Australian "Emergency Essence" are all useful.
See a professional if the attacks get worse; there may be a metabolic cause for these attacks.

DEPRESSION

Miserable, feeling down and withdrawn, lack of interest and meaning in the present. May have many dull aches and pains. Sufferers often manage to cope and keep going without realizing how depressed they are until something happens to point it out. If depression is prolonged, seek help.

Internal medicines
• St. John's wort for mild to moderate depression. Sage, fennel, rosemary.
• Add celery seed for aches and pains.

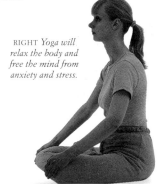

RIGHT *Yoga will relax the body and free the mind from anxiety and stress.*

LEFT *Inhale from a bottle of your favorite relaxing essential oil when you feel panicky.*

• Add valerian if associated with anxiety.
Other measures
• Massage and baths with uplifting essential oils: clary sage, rosemary, rose, lemon balm.
• Physical exercise releases anti-depressant chemicals into the brain, as does smiling.
• Flower remedies: gentian for depression from external cause, and mustard for depression arising suddenly with no cause.
(*See also Liver Disorders, p.122.*)

INSOMNIA

There are many causes of sleeplessness, including anxiety, depression, indigestion, over-excitement, and total exhaustion. People need less sleep as they get older (*see p.133*).

Internal medicines
Select herb according to cause.
• Valerian, skullcap, camomile, sage, peppermint, passionflower. Especially as a warm tea.
• For nightmares, try rosemary or wild thyme.
Other measures
• Lavender and hop pillows.
• Warm bath, ideally with lavender essential oil.
• No matter how late it is, take time to unwind or do some relaxing exercises before going to bed. Try reading or watching a video.
• The flower remedy white chestnut can stop unwanted internal chatter.

Herbalism in Pregnancy and Childbirth

During pregnancy the body must balance the needs of mother and baby. In general, herbal medicines are gentle remedies and well suited to problems that arise, although there are some that should not be taken (see below). Do not start any new treatment or herbal regime during the first three months of pregnancy, without consulting a professional in that field. Herbal treatment is best monitored by a professional herbalist throughout the pregnancy .

HERBAL STRATEGIES

- Nourishing.
- Relaxing.
- Using gentle remedies to deal with any symptoms.
- Preparing the womb for birth.
- Assisting labor.
- Recovery.

HERBS TO AVOID IN PREGNANCY

There are some herbs that should not be taken during pregnancy. These include: angelica, aloe leaf, comfrey, cinnamon, cloves, fennel, ginseng, lemon balm, marjoram, all mints, pennyroyal, parsley, sage, feverfew, golden seal, juniper, rue, wormwood, and strong laxatives. Avoid large doses of yarrow and cayenne.

Using herbs in cooking, in the normal way, is safe. If in doubt, consult a professional herbalist.

LEFT *Use gentle and nourishing herbs during pregnancy to prepare the body for birth.*

NOURISHMENT IN PREGNANCY

- Nettle tea and iron tonics.

Other measures

- A good, wholesome diet with plenty of fresh fruit and vegetables. Follow your body and eat what you feel you need, rather than following arbitrary advice. It is not necessary to drink milk as vegetables can provide enough calcium.
- If in doubt about the quality of your diet, buy a special formulation of vitamins and minerals for use in pregnancy. Avoid vitamin A supplements. It has now been proven that folic acid supplements reduce the risk of birth defects, including spina bifida, in the baby but they need to be taken from the start of the pregnancy, or preferably even before conception.

PREGNANCY SYMPTOMS

From the early months of pregnancy onward you may suffer from a variety of common complaints including:

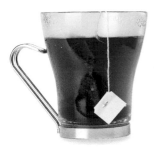

ABOVE *Drink raspberry tea for the last three months of pregnancy to assist labor.*

Nausea
• Ginger, marshmallow.
• If persistent, add dandelion.
• For morning sickness, keep a dry biscuit by the bed to eat before you get up.

Constipation
• Dandelion root, yellow dock.

Acid stomach
• Camomile, meadowsweet, marshmallow. Slippery elm drink.

High blood pressure
• Hawthorn or linden flowers and rest. Be sure to have your blood pressure monitored.

Stress and anxiety
• Camomile, linden flowers.

Varicose veins
• Marigold creams and lotions.

Vaginal thrush
• Live yogurt. Marigold pessaries or cream.

PREPARING FOR BIRTH

The healthier and fitter you are, the better your body will be able to cope with labor.
• Take raspberry leaf for the last three months.
• For the last two weeks, add two or three cloves to the tea or combine raspberry leaf and motherwort.

ASSISTING LABOR

Keep the following items in a special bag so that they are to hand. Be sure to inform the midwife or obstetrician about them.
• A large flask of your favorite relaxing tea, for example a mixture of camomile, linden flowers, and lemon balm.
• A bottle of massage oil containing relaxing and pain-killing oils for massage into the lower back during labor. A good combination is 20 drops each of clary sage, lavender, neroli, camomile, and clove oils in 3½fl oz (100ml) almond oil.
• A few pieces of Chinese ginseng to chew, for extra energy and to assist contractions when needed.

POSTNATAL RECOVERY

Discomfort for the first few days after birth is quite common. Skin tears or stitches can be extremely sore and painful.
• Marigold and comfrey to add to the bath.
• Marigold and comfrey cream for perineal tears.
• A tea of equal parts of raspberry leaf, St. John's wort, and camomile, drunk for a week or so after the birth, will aid quick recovery.

THE FIRST FEW WEEKS OF MOTHERHOOD

New mothers often wish they had known more of what to expect in childbirth, but no one can fully prepare you for the experience; it will be yours alone. Birth is the end of pregnancy and the beginning of a new task. It is a momentous time of confused emotions, which will swing from high to low spirits. Take time to adjust to your new situation. Ask for support from others.
• Vitex, raspberry leaf, fennel, and vervain.
If lowness or weepiness lasts longer than a few days, you may be suffering from depression – seek professional help.

BREAST-FEEDING

Not all mothers can breast-feed easily. Be sure to seek help if you have difficulties.
Breast massage (rubbing the breasts gently in small circles right up to the neck and round to the side, under the arms) will help prevent any congestion.
• Fennel or caraway tea to assist milk flow and reduce colic.
• Nettles, raspberry leaves, and marshmallow.
• Avoid sage as this tends to dry up breast milk.
• Cool compress of marigold will help sore nipples. The traditional compress of grated carrot is soothing and healing.

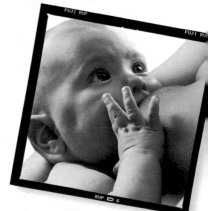

ABOVE *A marigold or cold carrot compress will help to soothe sore and tender nipples.*

Herbalism for Children

Childhood is a time of enormous growth and change. Children are constantly learning through play and experience, and need to be able to make mistakes in a safe environment. The rights of the child need to be defended: even though many children look and sometimes behave like adults from a very young age, it is important not to be deceived by outward appearances, but to give them the protection and care they still need. Make allowances for childish behavior: emotional development takes time.

REMEDIES FOR INFANTS

Infants learn from their parents, developing their appreciation of themselves from their attitude (positive or negative) to their experiences. If their parent is unsure, defensive, and fearful, the child will be too. Positive responses and encouragement will be strengthening and supportive.

Breast-feeding reduces the risk of all diseases. If there are allergies or food intolerances in the family, avoid cow's milk and other suspect foods until the child is one year old. Soy milk infant formulas are available if needed.

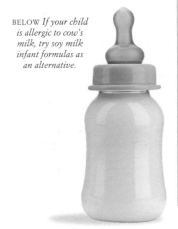

BELOW *If your child is allergic to cow's milk, try soy milk infant formulas as an alternative.*

COLIC

Colic is a severe stomach ache that occurs in babies from the age of 2–3 weeks and which usually disappears by three months. Babies who suffer from colic will often arch their backs and cry inconsolably.
• Add fennel, dill, caraway, or camomile tea to feeds or give to the mother if she is breast-feeding.

IRRITABILITY AND RESTLESSNESS

Find out the cause and respond appropriately. Babies give many subtle indications of precise need, and by careful observation you can learn your baby's own repertoire.
• General: camomile tea. Add 1–2 tsps (5–10ml) to feeds or 1–2 cups to the bathwater.
• Teething problems: add two cloves to a cup of camomile tea and use as above.
• Persistent sleeplessness: chop up the center of a romaine lettuce and simmer (not boil) for 5 minutes in a cup of breast milk or soy milk. Strain. Add a teaspoon of honey. Dosage: 2–3 tsp (10–15ml) before bed. Parents should also take relaxing herbs before bed so that, if they are woken, they can get back to sleep easily and quickly.
• Walnut flower remedy is good for clingy babies and at any time of change, such as weaning.

DIAPER RASH AND CRADLE CAP

Diaper rash is common among babies and can usually be avoided by changing the diaper frequently. Sometimes yellowy-brown crusts form on the baby's scalp. This is known as cradle cap.
• Use marigold ointment as an effective barrier cream for diaper rash, and marigold infused oil to soften and heal cradle cap.

DRY, ITCHY SKIN

Children's skin is particularly sensitive and skin reactions are a common problem in childhood. Young skin can often become dry and itchy, but responds well to herbal remedies.
• Marigold infused oil added to the bath. Marshmallow tea: 2–3 tsp (10–15ml) in feeds.

COLDS AND RUNNY NOSE

Viral infections are extremely common in children, particularly the first two years of life as they have little immunity to infection.
• Elderflower tea, 2–3 tsps (10–15ml) in feeds. Alternatively, put two or three cups in the bath.
• Eucalyptus essential oil in an oil burner at night.

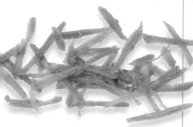

ABOVE *If your child has worms, add grated carrots to their daily meals.*

DIARRHEA

Diarrhea is characterized by the passing of loose and watery stools.
• Camomile and raspberry leaf tea with honey may be given freely by the teaspoonful.
• Carrot juice given freely.
• Rehydration mixture, available from a pharmacy.
See a professional if diarrhea is severe or if it persists for more than a day.

REMEDIES FOR CHILDREN

Children's illnesses have many factors – school, overexcitement, fear, or bullying may all contribute. Feigned "sickness" may be used as an avoidance technique or a demand for attention. With honesty and openness and it should be possible to help children meet challenges, so that they do not resort to "sickness."

CHILDREN'S FEVERS

A body temperature of over 100°F (38°C) indicates a fever.
• Try elderflowers, yarrow, linden flowers, catmint.
• Garlic honey to prevent colds and chest infections.
• Add marigold if the tonsils or lymph nodes ("glands") are swollen.
• Give echinacea and garlic for recurrent colds and fevers.

DIGESTIVE UPSETS

Encourage children to enjoy new foods and tastes, but never force them to eat anything they do not like. A baby should join family meals as soon as possible. Many of the social skills we need are learned at the table.
• Camomile, catmint.
• Add meadowsweet if there is a fever.

CONSTIPATION

Infrequent (less than one bowel movement every three to four days) or difficult bowel movement.
• Prune juice, syrup of figs.
• Senna syrup if necessary, but only for a few days at a time.

INTESTINAL WORMS

Itchy bottom, worse at night. Look out for the worms or eggs in the stools. Very common among children. The eggs are difficult to kill, so look out for a recurrence of the symptoms.
• Garlic honey, 2–4 tsps (10–20ml) before breakfast for two weeks.
• Thyme tea.
• Grated carrots daily.
Other measures
• Wash hands well before meals.
• Change bedding and nightwear frequently.

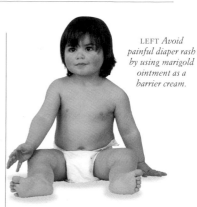

LEFT *Avoid painful diaper rash by using marigold ointment as a barrier cream.*

HEAD LICE

Itchy scalp. Look out for the lice or their eggs, which stick to the hair. Very common in school children, and not a sign of poor hygiene. The whole family should be treated.
• Tea tree essential oil: add 5–10 drops to the rinsing water after washing the hair. This can also be used as a preventive regime.
• Quassia wood chips: make a strong decoction and use it to rinse the hair after washing. This is a good preventive regime.

BED-WETTING

• St. John's wort, horsetail, marshmallow, thyme, mullein.
Other measures
• No drinks in the evening. Make sure the child empties the bladder before bed. If due to heavy sleeping, take the child to the lavatory again after 2 hours. Don't scold.

CAUTION

Always check with a medical professional to make sure that a fever is not life-threatening, before treating at home.

Herbalism for the Elderly

The definition of old age has changed as our expectations, length, and quality
of life have improved. In humoral terms, the dominant element is phlegm:
old age is phlegmatic. The benefits of this are being steady and reliable, solid but
not fixed, more flexible than when middle-aged, and less liable to fly off the
handle than younger people. It can still be a period of good health and vitality
if you have previously taken good care of yourself.

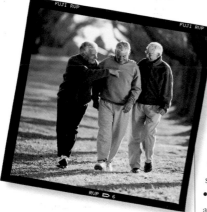

LEFT *The elderly will*
benefit greatly from
some form of regular
gentle exercise.

• Cayenne for feelings of cold with lethargy and weaknesses. Use a tincture or vinegar extract. Dosage: 4 or 5 drops in a little warm water or herbal tea three to six times daily.
• Yarrow is good for varicose veins and cold feet.

Heart
• Hawthorn for "heart failure" with breathlessness on exertion, blue lips, and swollen ankles. Two or three cups daily. Added cayenne is also helpful.
• Add motherwort for racing and irregular heart beat.
• Add ginkgo for improving circulation to the brain and for varicose veins.

CIRCULATION
The circulation tends to become weaker in old age. In traditional terms elderly people get "colder" and require more warming remedies. An extra layer of clothing, frequent warm and "warming" drinks, a regular form of exercise, and warm foot baths are both excellent and extremely cheap ways of putting heat into their body.

General
• Rosemary as a long-term herb to support circulation and treat symptoms such as aches and pains that are worse in cold, damp weather. Dosage: one or two cups of the infusion daily.

DIGESTION
As we age and become less active, digestion tends to slow down and the absorption of vitamins and minerals is decreased. We still need regular, four-hourly, good-quality nourishment, however, but meals may be smaller.

Remedies for general improvement of digestion and absorption.
• Cayenne. Dose as above.
• Angelica, elecampane.
Remedies rich in minerals and vitamins (*see specific entry for indications*).
• Kelp, nettles, horsetail, and oats.
For constipation (may follow from eating less).
• Chinese angelica, dandelion root, yellow dock.
• Aloe vera gel or the leaf tincture, which is stronger.
• Cleansing "wake-up" drink each morning; fruit or rosemary vinegar in water is a favorite.

CAUTION

As metabolism slows down, remedies stay in the system for longer, and smaller doses are required. Very weak, elderly people should take half the ordinary adult dose.

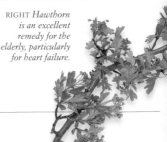

RIGHT *Hawthorn*
is an excellent
remedy for the
elderly, particularly
for heart failure.

Other measures

• Add gentle spices to food: cinnamon, ginger, fennel seed.

• In general eat a high-fiber diet including greens and whole grains. For acute attacks of pain, decrease fiber content for a short while and eat white bread (originally made to rest the guts) and root vegetables.

• Simply drinking more (especially water in the morning) will often relieve constipation.

FATIGUE AND LOW ENERGY

Warming tonics for maintaining strength, sexual energy, and vitality.

• Sage, Chinese ginseng, burdock root, and saw palmetto (*Serenoa serrulata*).

A tonic tea, melissa or sage and honey, every morning is an excellent routine for tiredness.

MEMORY LOSS, CONFUSION, ANXIETY

Forgetfulness and confusion are common traits of old age as the mind as well as the body deteriorates. This is commonly accompanied by anxiety, depression, and mood swings.

• Sage, lemon balm (*Melissa officinalis*), mugwort, Siberian ginseng are all worth taking.

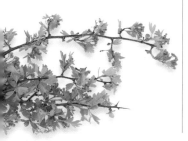

• Ginkgo if accompanied by dizziness. Also for the first stages of Alzheimer's disease.

Other measures

• Adult education classes and study. The brain will work better when it is exercised.

• Add oats to the diet.

• "Brain food," including oily fish (salmon, sardines, mackerel), four portions a week.

SLEEP PROBLEMS

As the body ages it needs less sleep. If you adapt your expectations, you may find that you can enjoy a new hobby for the extra hours. Many retired people develop a pattern of cat naps or an afternoon rest, together with only four to five hours night sleep.

Insomnia

• Lavender and hop pillows.

• Lavender baths and warm drinks are especially helpful.

• (*See Nervous System, pp. 126–7.*)

EYESIGHT

It is inadvisable to put drops into the eye without professional guidance. Eye exercises, and head and neck massage are extremely useful to maintain blood circulation to the eyes.

Internal remedies

• Burdock seed heads, mugwort, bilberry jam (preferably sugar free).

• Carrots and carrot juice strengthen the eyes.

• Foods containing Vitamin C also promote clearness of vision.

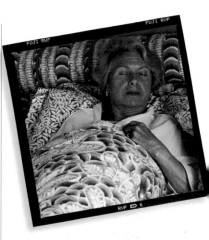

ABOVE *Herbs, such as lavender, can be used to help those who have difficulty sleeping.*

TERMINAL CARE

The dying process, like the process of any other experience, can be a full and fulfilling one. People make choices throughout their lives that determine the manner and time of their death, choices to be honored and respected. Pain can be controlled with orthodox treatment, and herbs can be used to ease other symptoms. Washing with camomile tea or lavender water is soothing. Compresses and foot or hand baths are appreciated. Comfrey and lavender ointment is good for bed sores. Liberal use of marigold tea and Rescue Remedy helps the carer and the patient, equally, to let go with dignity.

The Medicine Chest and First Aid

The aim of a medicine chest is to have on hand the items needed for meeting your family's everyday health needs. It is in addition to a first-aid box. Responding promptly and accurately to illness will shorten its duration and prevent it getting worse. The contents of the chest will depend on the ages and general state of health of all the members of the household, so before stocking it, make notes on the kinds of minor illnesses that recur in your family.

If you have children you will probably need a cough syrup, a tea for "summer tummy," and a large bottle of calendula tincture for all the inevitable small cuts and bruises. Select the herbs and decide on the amount you will require for a course of treatment. A 2oz (50g) bag of thyme will see an average family through the year (one upset tummy and two chesty coughs), although a 4oz (125g) bag might be needed if the thyme is to be added to a tonic remedy for a family that is susceptible to minor infections.

Replace herbs yearly to retain their freshness. Keep the medicine chest in a cool place, out of the reach of children. None of the herbs are poisonous as such, but a small child can become very sick from the alcohol in a bottle of tincture.

The medicine chest should also include a notebook. This will enable you to keep a check on the stock, make notes of the remedies and recipes, note what works and what does not. This knowledge will be invaluable to you, and will also make a priceless gift of knowledge to pass on to your children. (In the 17th century, each grand house had a book in which to keep the recipes of everyday life.)

HERBS AND REMEDIES FOR THE MEDICINE CHEST

The following herbs are invaluable additions to the medicine chest.

• Soothing, cooling, healing salve – comfrey ointment.
• Antiseptic and cooling tincture – calendula tincture. Use diluted for compresses.
• Laxative – fig syrup; dock herb.
• Digestive – peppermint; fennel.
• Sedative – camomile; linden.
• For a muscle relaxant and joint warmer – use camomile, ginger, and thyme infused oil for massage. Also cramp bark for internal use.
• Cough syrup – thyme and coltsfoot honey.
• Cough syrup and lung antiseptic – garlic honey.
• Female tea – parsley, sage, and camomile tea.
• Sore throat, mouth and gum problems – sage tea. Strong sage tea as gargle.

More specific remedies can be bought or made in response to need.

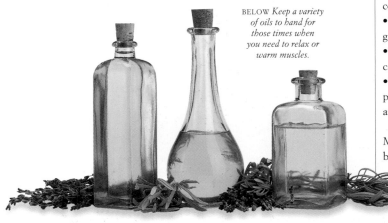

BELOW *Keep a variety of oils to hand for those times when you need to relax or warm muscles.*

FIRST AID

First aid is simple to learn and can be life-saving. It is the most important aspect of home healthcare, and learning how to deal with a medical emergency should be a priority for everyone. Many schools and other organizations run first-aid classes, and proper training will enable you to act quickly, confidently, and responsibly.

All households should have a first-aid box to hand for emergencies. The box should include small scissors, tweezers, measuring spoons, an eye bath, thermometer, lint, small plasters, cotton bandages of different sizes, a large crepe bandage, and adhesive tape. To maintain sterility, the dressings should be unopened.

The first aid box should also contain:
• Calendula tincture for cuts, wounds, and compresses.
• Lavender essential oil for burns (once the burn has been sufficiently cooled).
• A flower remedy for shock. Bach, Healing Herbs, and Australian Essences all make a shock remedy.

KITCHEN REMEDIES

The average kitchen contains several invaluable remedies. Salt, pepper, lemon, honey, and garlic are found in almost all kitchens. These are fine remedies in their own right, and skillful use of them can provide initial treatment for many conditions and complaints.

Salt – use a weak salt solution, the strength of tears, to clean wounds, as a gargle, and to bathe eyes. A salt bath (1–2 cups per bath) is useful for stiffness and after infections to clear the system.

Pepper is a warming stimulant. Cayenne pepper is best, but a small pinch of any pepper in a herbal tea will help prevent chills when damp and cold.

Lemon juice in hot water with a pinch of pepper and a spoonful of honey is a traditional cold and flu remedy. It should be taken at the first sniffle, then freely. (*See Cayenne, p. 88.*)

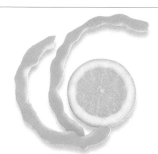

ABOVE *An infusion of lemon and water will help cool the body in times of fever.*

Lemon – the weak acid of lemon juice with water helps cool the system and can be drunk freely for fevers and in some cases of cystitis. Lemon peel can be rubbed on the skin as a treatment for fungal infections.

Honey is a popular and soothing antiseptic for children's coughs. It can also be used locally for itchy, dry skin conditions.

Garlic and onion may be used internally and externally as an antiseptic, as an expectorant, and also for drawing. (*See Garlic, pp.36–37.*)

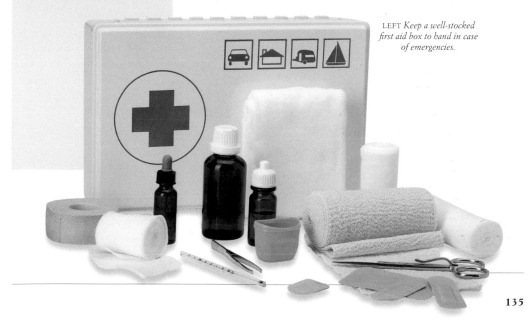

LEFT *Keep a well-stocked first aid box to hand in case of emergencies.*

Visiting a Herbalist

The herbal remedies described in the Materia Medica are safe for use at home, but they are only a small part of the pharmacy of nature. Herbs can complement other treatments or offer a complete alternative. In the hands of a skilled and responsible practitioner, herbs are powerful and potent medicines.

A CONSULTANT MEDICAL HERBALIST

Personal recommendation remains the best way to find a practitioner. However, if you do not know anyone who is able to recommend a good herbalist, ask one of the organizations that keep a register of qualified practitioners. For a list of these refer to Useful Addresses at the end of the book (*see p. 138*).

Sometimes herbal practitioners are seen as the call of last resort, to be consulted when all other searches for a cure or remedy are exhausted. However, this is not the best time to visit a herbalist or a fair trial of herbal medicine. It is much better to go at the first sign of a problem – herbalists can treat both chronic and acute conditions. You can register with a herbalist in the same way as with a primary healthcare physician, or general practitioner. The whole family may register and use herbal medicine for all their ailments.

THE FIRST CONSULTATION

The first consultation will last approximately an hour and address all aspects of your health and lifestyle. There may be a physical examination, and blood pressure and urine tests. As with a physician, rapport and trust is important. If you do not feel comfortable, or feel that you are not being heard, find another herbalist. A good relationship should last for life. If the herbalist cannot help, you will be referred to another specialist.

It is important that the herbalist knows all that you are taking, so take any other medicine with you, including orthodox medicine. The herbalist will know about herb/drug interactions, and will use this information when formulating a prescription. Treatment will include herbs in various forms, as well as advice on diet, health management, and lifestyle.

All herbal remedies are specific to the individual; do not give your medicine to others. Take them as prescribed for the full course. This may be some months in chronic conditions.

DURATION OF TREATMENT

Follow-up visits usually take place after two to eight weeks, depending on the type, severity, and disposition of the condition. Most conditions, even serious chronic conditions, can be helped to some degree or another and the health improved. Chronic conditions may need six or more months' treatment, although a general improvement should be felt within three. Acute conditions may respond immediately.

You may wish to inform your orthodox physician about the visit, or you may prefer the herbalist to write. This is up to you. The herbalist will respect your wishes. All consultations are held in the strictest confidence.

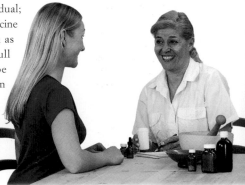

RIGHT *It is important to have a good relationship with your herbalist.*

CASE HISTORY

Jack, 5 year-old boy, just starting school. Over the past two years has taken six courses of antibiotics to ease a series of stubborn colds and ear infections. Mother worried that illness will affect school attendance. Grommets recommended by doctor. Mother wishes to try herbal medicine before making the decision.

Tincture
Elderflower tincture 5 tsp (25ml)
Echinacea tincture 5 tsp (25ml)
Poke root tincture ½ tsp (2ml)
Honey 60ml
Shake well before use.
Dosage: 1 tsp (5ml), three times day.
Strategy: to strengthen immune system, reducing susceptibility to infection. To clear ear through lymphatic system.

Cold and Flu Tea
Dried elderflowers 1 part
Dried peppermint leaf 1 part
Dried yarrow leaf and flower 1 part
Make as tea for whole family at first sign of cold symptoms. Drink freely.

Room spray
Water 2½ cups (600ml)
Eucalyptus essential oil 5 drops
Lavender essential oil 5 drops
To humidify centrally heated house, use a room spray. Spray bedroom and living area regularly.
Strategy: to maintain health of nasal mucosa, and prevent it drying out (child tends to breathe through mouth while asleep).

Result
First winter: one cold treated with flu tea and chest rub. Generally healthier and enjoying school.

CASE HISTORY

Ruth, single mother aged 26, two children aged seven and four. P.M.S., breast pain, bloating, irritability, temper, exhaustion, depression. Whole lifestyle dominated by children's needs. Sometimes too stressed or tired to eat all day.

Diet. Must eat little and often. Carbohydrate every 4 hours.

General supportive tea
Dried camomile flowers 1 part
Dried lemon balm leaf and flower 1 part
Dried parsley leaf 1 part
Make as tea. Honey may be added.
Dosage: 2–3 cups day.
Strategy: to reduce overall stress, raise spirits, clear water retention.

Vitex tincture
10 tsp (50ml) in dropper bottle
Dosage:15 drops a day after ovulation (14 days after menstruation) until period starts.
For three months.
Strategy: to rebalance hormonal interactions.

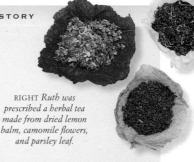

RIGHT *Ruth was prescribed a herbal tea made from dried lemon balm, camomile flowers, and parsley leaf.*

Result
First period was little better, although breasts were noticeably less tender.
Each period improved until patient announced herself better after fourth cycle.
Enrolled on training course to begin when youngest starts school.

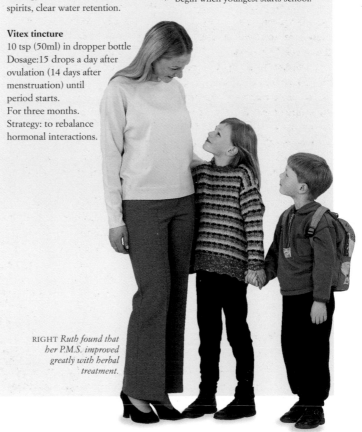

RIGHT *Ruth found that her P.M.S. improved greatly with herbal treatment.*

Useful Addresses

For general information on all aspects of herbs and herbalism.

U.K.

British Herbal Medicine Association
Sun House
Church Street
Stroud
Gloucester
GL5 1JL

The Herb Society
Deddington Hill Farm
Warmington
Banbury
OX17 1XB

The Natural Medicines Group
P.O. Box 5
Ilkeston
Derbyshire
DE7 8LX

U.S.A.

The Herb Quarterly
Box 548 MH
Boiling Springs
PA 17007

AUSTRALIA

The Australian Herb Society
PO Box 110
Mapleton 4560

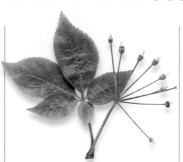

INTERNET

The internet now has many pages maintained by herbal professionals, general associations, growers, producers, and retailers

http://sunsite.unc.edu/herbmed/
Gives access to FAQ archives for news:alt.folklore.herbs,

In the U.K. a good place to start is the Home page of the "Herb Society [U.K.]."

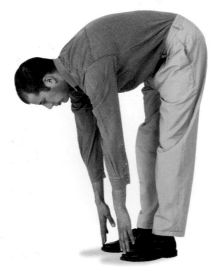

SUPPLIERS

The first option should be to look for high quality locally grown herbs. There are many small growers and tincture/remedy makers throughout the world producing a high quality and ethical product. Mail order is available if this is impossible. Check local directories and the Internet.

Where to find a professional herbalist
The following organizations keep lists of registered and qualified herbal practitioners. Always send a S.S.A.E. when seeking information.

U.K.

The General Council and Register of Consultant Herbalists
32 King Edward Road
Swansea
SA1 4LL

The National Institute of Medical Herbalists
56 Longbrook Street
Exeter
Devon
EX4 6AH

U.S.A.

The American Herbalists Guild
PO Box 1683
Soquel
CA 95073

AUSTRALIA

The National Herbalist Association of Australia
PO Box 65
Kingsgrove
N.S.W. 2208

Victoria Herbalists Association
24 Russell Street
Northcote
Victoria 3070

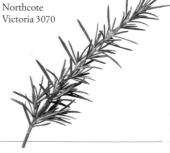

Further Reading

GENERAL

BARTRAM, THOMAS, *Encyclopaedia of Herbal Medicine*, Grace Publishers, 1995.

BROOKE, ELIZABETH, *A Woman's Book of Herbs*, The Women's Press Ltd., 1991.

CHEVALIER, ANDREW, *Encyclopedia of Medicinal Plants*, Dorling Kindersley, 1993.

DAWSON, ADELE G., *Herbs Partners in Life: A Guide to Cooking, Gardening and Healing with Wild and Cultivated Plants*, Healing Arts Press, 1991.

FORSTER, STEPHE, AND YUE, C., *Herbal Emissaries*, Healing Arts Press, 1992.

GREEN, JAMES, *The Male Herbal: Health Care for Men and Boys*, The Crossing Press, 1991.

HEDLEY, CHRISTOPHER, AND SHAW, NON, *Herbal Remedies: A Practical Beginner's Guide to Making Effective Remedies in the Kitchen*, Parragon, 1996.

HOFFMAN, DAVID, *The Complete Illustrated Holistic Herbal*, Element, 1996.

MCINTYRE, ANNE, *Herbs for Pregnancy and Childbirth*, Sheldon Press, 1988.

ODY, PENNY, *The Herb Society's Complete Medicinal Herbal*, Dorling Kindersley, 1993, 1996.

VYIDERT, MELLIE, *The Psychic Garden: Plants and their Esoteric Relationship with Man*, Thorsons, 1980.

WOOD, MATTHEW, *Seven Herbs: Plants as Teachers*, North Atlantic Books, 1988.

REFERENCE

BLAMEY, MARJORIE, AND GREY-WILSON, CHRISTOPHER, *The Illustrated Flora of Britain and Northern Europe*, Domino Books/Hodder and Stoughton, 1989.

British Herbal Pharmacopoeia, British Herbal Medicine Association,1971. Reprinted 1987.

GRIEVES, MAUDE, EDITED BY MRS C. F. LEYEL, *A Modern Herbal*, Jonathan Cape, 1931.

MILLS, SIMON Y., *Out of the Earth: The Essential Book of Herbal Medicine*, Penguin Books, 1991.

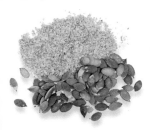

HISTORY

Culpeper's Complete Herbal, Wordsworth Editions Ltd., 1995.

GRIGGS, BARBARA, *Green Pharmacy: A History of Herbal Medicine*, Jill Norman & Hobhouse, 1981.

ROHDE, ELEANOR SINCLAIR, *The Old English Herbals*, Minerva Press,1922. Reprinted in paperback.

RATTI, OSCAR, AND WESTBROOK ADELE, (TRS.), *The Medieval Health Handbook*, George Braziller Inc.,1976.

STREHLOW, DR. WIGHARD, AND HERTZKA, GOTTFRIED, M.D., *Hildegard of Bingen's Medicine*, Bear and Company, 1988.

GARDENING

GARDINER, ANTHONY, *A Garden Herbal*, Sunburst Books, 1995.

STICKLAND, SUE, *Planning your Organic Herb Garden*, Thorsons, 1986.

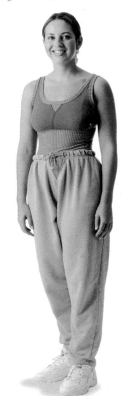

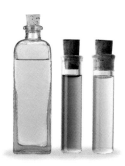

Glossary

Acute. A sudden and short illness, for example, flu or tonsillitis. Long-term illnesses (see chronic) may have acute phases where the condition is more active, as in arthritis.

Adaptogen. Helps the body deal with stress. For example, Siberian ginseng.

Allopathic. The homeopathic term of reference for conventional medicine.

Alterative. Corrects disordered bodily functions. For example, parsley, yellow dock.

Analgesic. Has the effect of relieving pain. For example, willow, clove, camomile.

Anaphrodisiac. Diminishes excessive sexual desire. For example, willow bark.

Antiemetic. Settles the stomach and prevents sickness. For example, ginger.

Anti-inflammatory. Reduces inflammations. For example, willow, cabbage, camomile.

Antiseptic. Kills bacteria and prevents infection. For example, thyme, garlic, honey. Most essential oils.

Antispasmodic. Alleviates spasms and cramp. For example, camomile, ginger, fennel, cramp bark.

Astringent. Drying, contracting, and reducing secretions. For example; raspberry leaf, witch hazel.

Bitter. A bitter quality that stimulates appetite and promotes digestion. For example, camomile, dandelion, dock.

Carminative. Relaxes the stomach and clears wind. For example, peppermint, fennel, cinnamon.

Cholagogue. Promotes free flow of bile. For example, dandelion root, dock.

Chronic. A long-standing illness such as arthritis. Chronic ailments need time and management to improve.

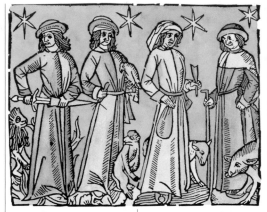

Circulatory stimulant. Warms and promotes circulation. For example, cayenne.

Compress. An application of crushed fresh herbs or lint soaked in tea or tincture, used to relieve pain or swelling. For example, cabbage, camomile, marigold.

Decoction. An extract of herbs made by boiling in water, Usually used for root and barks.

Decongestant. Relieves congestion in nose and sinuses. For example, peppermint, horseradish, rosemary.

Demulcent. Soothes irritation. For example, marshmallow, comfrey, honey.

Diaphoretic. Induces sweating. For example, hot sage, cayenne, elderflower.

Digestive. Promotes good digestion. For example, camomile, ginger, oats, rosemary.

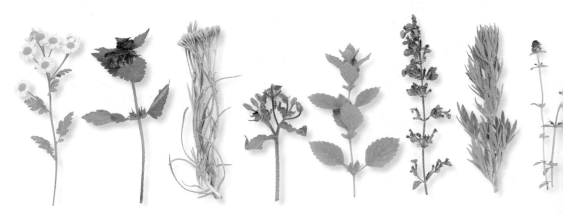

Diuretic. Promotes urination. For example, dandelion leaf and root, parsley.

Drawing. Draws poisons from boils and abscesses. For example, oats, marshmallow, honey.

Emetic. Promotes vomiting. For example, salt, mustard, meadowsweet in large doses.

Emmenagogue. Promotes menstruation. For example, mugwort, peppermint, sage. Emmenagogs should not be taken in pregnancy.

Emollient. Softening and soothing skin preparations. For example, mallow.

Expectorant. Helps expel mucus from the lungs. For example, thyme, garlic.

Febrifuge. Helps to reduce fevers and lower temperature. For example, yarrow, camomile, sage.

Fomentation. A hot compress. Lint soaked in warm herb tea/tincture. Used to warm, and relieve pain and cold stiffness. For example, camomile, oats, marigold.

Fungicide. For fungal infestations. For example, aloes, garlic, marigold.

Hepatic. Strengthens the liver. For example, dandelion, turmeric, thyme, rosemary.

Infusion. Soaking a herb in hot or cold water to make a tea, or oil to make a rub.

Laxative. Promotes bowel movement. For example, dock, dandelion root, senna.

Liniments. Warming rubs usually made by mixing tinctures and herbal infused oil.

Lymphatic deobstructant. Promotes proper lymphatic function. For "swollen glands" and chronic infection. For example, marigold.

Mucilage. A substance containing gelatinous constituents that are demulcent.

Nervine. Restoring and strengthening the nervous system. For example, camomile, St. John's wort, lemon balm (Melissa).

Poultice. A thickened application, usually made by mixing herbal extract into a demulcent base such as slippery elm powder, Usually applied warm. Used to relieve pain or draw abscesses.

Psychotropic. The effect of drugs that alter the state of mind.

Relaxant. Relaxes tension in the body. For example, camomile.

Restorative. Strengthen and promotes well-being after illness. For example, hawthorn, dandelion, linden.

Rubefacient. A local irritant that causes reddening on the skin. For example, cayenne, mustard, sage essential oil.

Sedative. Calms the nerves. For example, camomile, linden, clove.

Stimulant. Increases activity. For example, cayenne, coffee, ginseng.

Styptic. Stems blood flow. For example, yarrow.

Tincture. An extract of herbs made by soaking in alcohol and water.

Tonic. Strengthens and enlivens whole, or part, of the body. For example, general tonic – sage, verbena.

Digestive tonic – rosemary, camomile.

Nerve tonic – linden, St. John's wort, lemon balm (Melissa).

Blood tonic – nettle.

Vermifuge. Kills worms and intestinal parasites. For example, wormwood, thyme, garlic.

141

Index

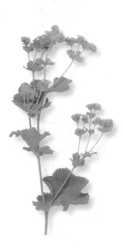

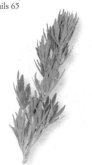

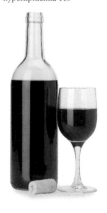

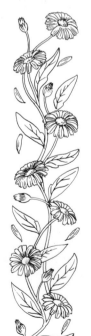

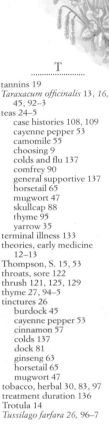

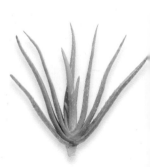